Successful Learning in Pharmacy

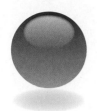

Successful Learning in Pharmacy

Developing Study and Communication Skills

Parastou Donyai

Daniel Grant

Nilesh Patel

Reading School of Pharmacy

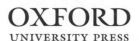

OXFORD

UNIVERSITY PRESS

OXFORD
UNIVERSITY PRESS

Great Clarendon Street, Oxford, OX2 6DP,
United Kingdom

Oxford University Press is a department of the University of Oxford.
It furthers the University's objective of excellence in research, scholarship,
and education by publishing worldwide. Oxford is a registered trade mark of
Oxford University Press in the UK and in certain other countries

First edition 2017

Impression: 1

Published in the United States of America by Oxford University Press
198 Madison Avenue, New York, NY 10016, United States of America

British Library Cataloguing in Publication Data
Data available

Library of Congress Control Number: 2017932603

ISBN 978-0-19-964211-3

Printed in Great Britain by
Bell & Bain Ltd., Glasgow

Overview of contents

Contents in full

Preface

One September as the start of a new academic year was fast approaching and I looked forward to welcoming new pharmacy undergraduates to the department, it occurred to me how useful it would be to capture in one place all the advice I was about to give so that the students could access the right information again and again, as and when needed. Imagine then the serendipity when Jonathan Crowe and his team at Oxford University Press contacted me at the exact same time to talk about pharmacy books. The conversation gave rise to the idea of a communication and study skills book written specifically to cater for the unique and important needs of pharmacy students. In the months that followed, we sketched out a template for the book and were delighted when two other academic pharmacist colleagues based at Reading School of Pharmacy, Dan Grant and Nilesh Patel, joined the writing team.

A guide to the book

University learning is a new experience for most pharmacy students, who, like you, want to know what to expect from a degree course and, importantly, how to personalize and maximize their learning while at university; this is the theme of **Chapter 1**. Lectures are new to the majority of pharmacy students so **Chapter 2** focuses on how to get the best from lectures while recognizing your preferred learning style. Pharmacy is a science-based degree; with this in mind, **Chapter 3** is all about learning in the laboratory. It discusses how to carry out experiments safely, explores the basis of scientific enquiry, and considers how you gather data and present that data in your lab report.

Whether writing a report, an essay, or basically engaging in any learning activity, you will invariably need to access new information, for example to help bolster your understanding or demonstrate your familiarity with existing literature. **Chapter 4** gives a thorough explanation of the different relevant sources of information for pharmacy and how to search and access these. **Chapter 5** then concentrates on writing essays, something you might do as coursework or in an exam. It explores how to interpret the essay question, how to structure and compose your essay, and how to write in your own words, appropriately referencing material you have used in your writing.

In addition to written exams, you will also encounter verbal assessments in your pharmacy course; **Chapter 6** provides tips for success in designing and delivering poster presentations, performing in oral examinations, and preparing for a specific type of assessment where your knowledge is put to the test in a series of stations.

The academic demands placed on you will increase in the latter years of your pharmacy course as the complexity and depth of learning you will be expected to achieve, and your independence as a learner, increase. With this in mind, the second half of this book focuses on higher-level skills. **Chapter 7** explores reading and thinking with a critical mind, and writing with a critical voice. To progress successfully through your degree, you will, of course, have to sit a range of written exams, and so **Chapter 8** describes effective revision plans, tips for managing pre-exam stress, and strategies for taking exams, as well as reviewing example question formats.

Learning pharmacy involves a great deal of working with others. **Chapter 9** focuses on professionalism, communication skills, team working, interprofessional learning, and different group-based learning activities. Many of the skills covered in **Chapter** 9 of course relate to the practice of pharmacy, your future career, and will therefore help with your employability.

A UK-based pharmacy course will provide you with the opportunity to attend pharmacy practice placements. **Chapter 10** is all about engaging with and learning from a practice workplace, as well as sourcing additional pharmacy training posts. When you are working in a pharmacy your role will often involve the use of current best evidence to make decisions about the care of patients. **Chapter 11** therefore focuses on the different types of clinical evidence and how to evaluate these types of data to answer specific clinical questions. Pharmacists continue to learn well into their retirement. This continuing professional development (CPD) is the focus of the final chapter of this book, **Chapter 12**, which introduces the CPD cycle, and guides you to start your own lifelong learning journey.

Learning from this book

This book uses a range of learning features.

- **Learning outcomes** open each chapter and set out what you should achieve having studied from each chapter.
- **Key points** at the end of each chapter summarize the main points covered—a useful tool at revision time.
- **Annotated examples** of good and bad practice, and **tips** and **checklists** throughout, provide pointers for making your learning as effective as possible, while avoiding common issues and pitfalls.
- Student-based and patient-based **case studies** illustrate the reality of various key concepts and ideas.
- Example **exam questions** and **answers** give you a flavour of the kind of assessment you are likely to encounter during your studies to help you prepare.
- **Further reading** and **references** are provided to take your learning one step further.

We have written this book to guide you right from the beginning of your degree through to the final years, and hope you will find it a refreshing and helpful companion to your pharmacy studies. Put simply, there is no other book available to cover the material we have carefully constructed for your use here. We sincerely hope you enjoy using this book—and wish you well in your future pharmacy careers.

Parastou Donyai
Reading
August 2016

Acknowledgements

I thank Jonathan Crowe for supporting this project through his detailed guidance and his continued patience and encouragement. I thank my family for their unquestioning support of the many projects, including this one, that seep into our private lives. This book is dedicated to students who find meaning in Simone de Beauvoir's words: 'One is not born a genius, one becomes a genius'.

  Parastou Donyai

Firstly, I would like to thank Parastou Donyai for the opportunity to contribute to this book. For me, helping write this book has been a new and unique learning experience. Whatever stage of your life you are at, learning never stops. Secondly, I would also like to thank Jonathan Crowe and his team at Oxford University Press for their support and guidance.

  Nilesh Patel

I would like to thank Parastou Donyai for giving me the opportunity to join her on the journey of writing this book, and Jonathan Crowe for his support and guidance along the way. It has been a new and interesting challenge, and a fantastic learning experience. I dedicate my chapters to my family and friends, and pharmacy students past and present, who keep me constantly learning and aiming to be the best I can be.

  Daniel Grant

1

Learning to learn at university

 Overview

We invite you to read this chapter in its entirety, especially if you are in the early stages of your pharmacy degree—we have brought together a range of crucial information essential to university learning. Whatever your stage of learning, we are sure you will find something in this chapter to bolster your knowledge and understanding. During this chapter, we are going to explain the experience of being at university so that you can better prepare for the challenges that lie ahead. This chapter will examine what you should expect specifically from the people who will teach you and what, in return, they will expect from you. This will lead to the concept of personalized learning and how to develop skills that will help you get the most from your university experience. The chapter will look at the aims of a pharmacy degree and the way in which pharmacy is taught and assessed, and will examine, among other topics, the values and attitudes expected of pharmacy students.

 Learning outcomes

You should be able to demonstrate knowledge and understanding of the following after working through this chapter:

- what to expect from a pharmacy degree course at university;
- how to personalize and maximize your learning experience at university.

Learn what to expect at university

One feature that unifies all undergraduate pharmacy students is that you will be studying a full-time course which requires a full-time commitment. Beyond this unifying feature, however, there is no such thing as a 'typical' pharmacy student. You might have a part-time job to support your learning (but you would need to be careful about the impact of this on your studies); you could feasibly be a mature student making a career change; or you might have just turned 18 and be starting university having always wanted to do pharmacy. You might be financially supported by your family or you might have a family of your own with associated financial concerns; you could be living at home with your parents or you could be some distance away from them in halls of residence. You might have even deferred your entry onto the course as you accrued sufficient funds needed for a full-time commitment to studying pharmacy.

Pharmacy attracts a range of students with different upbringings, personal and social circumstances, preferences, and obligations. But whatever your background and ongoing concerns, you will have one major issue in common with everybody else on your course. This is that you will first need to learn how to become a pharmacy student. In this process, you will make new relationships and might alter your existing social networks. You will need to negotiate your way around a new geographical and virtual space; and, most significantly, you will have to learn how to interact with your tutors and lecturers and develop study habits for a completely new learning environment. Some students find this shift to the university setting particularly challenging. Even those who have attended university previously (e.g. to study a science degree) can face specific challenges as they adjust to a course that emphasizes communication skills and application of knowledge to real-life situations. You can, of course, prepare and help yourself for a smooth transition to becoming a pharmacy student, as explained below.

Becoming a pharmacy student

Firstly, you have to recognize that university is very different to school, college, or other learning institutions you have previously experienced. It is important, therefore, not to solely rely on those experiences to inform your understanding of the culture of university. Unless you were part of a school–university partnership then you will quickly find that university is entirely different to anything you would have experienced before. At university, you are expected to become an independent learner. This means taking on full responsibility for your day-to-day activities, as well as medium- to long-term plans for learning your subject and interacting with others. Secondly, you have to accept that whatever your expectations are, even after reading this chapter, nothing will replace the knowledge you will gain from ultimately experiencing the university life that your particular setting has to offer.

On accepting these two conditions, we can move on to define some of the general values and rules that will help you acclimatize to the experience of being a pharmacy student at university. The focus will be on academic staff, what to expect from them, and what they expect from you.

Understanding who teaches pharmacy

One of the important distinctions between school and university is the role of the teacher (we will call them academics from now on) in your learning. A variety of people are likely to teach pharmacy at your university, including professors and lecturers, teacher-practitioners and teaching fellows, research staff and doctoral students (PhD students), technicians, and even others. Some lectures might be delivered by those based outside of your school of pharmacy. The range of job titles you will encounter will depend on which university you attend; some of the most common job titles are listed in Box 1.1. Of course, professors are more senior to lecturers, but staff grades can be interpreted differently, depending on the convention used by your university.

The important thing to note is that although traditional academics (lecturers and professors) normally spend most of their working hours at the university, they also typically have an obligation to conduct research on top of their teaching. This is especially so of some academics who are given a remit to focus on research. This competing commitment can make it

Box 1.1 The range of staff likely to teach pharmacy at university

Academic staff:

Lecturers/senior lecturers/principal lecturers

Readers

Associate professors/professors

Academics, on the whole, will be tasked with teaching, research, and organizational responsibilities. They will act as tutors and heads of divisions and departments.

Teaching-focused staff:

Teacher-practitioners

Clinical lecturers*

Teaching fellows

Teaching-focused staff will be tasked with teaching and organizational tasks. They might act as tutors and also supervise research projects and give placement support.

* Some devote 50% of time to research.

Research staff:

Doctoral students (PhD students)

Post-doctoral students

Research assistants/associates/fellows

Research staff will be tasked with a research project or other research duties. They will become involved in some teaching activities for their career development.

Support staff:

Technicians

Demonstrators

Administrators

Support staff, on the whole, will be tasked with assisting academics and teaching-focused staff with their responsibilities. Technicians can be research or teaching focused, depending on their role.

difficult for students to access some academics outside of scheduled teaching hours—a factor that is important for you to understand and work around, meaning we have devoted a separate paragraph subheaded 'Contacting academics if you need help' to explain lecturer contact.

You may also be taught by teaching fellows; these are normally people employed on a full-time basis at the university but who have a focus on teaching with little involvement in research. Teacher-practitioners and clinical lecturers are normally registered pharmacists who will work in a patient-facing pharmacy practice setting when not teaching at the university. Some teaching practitioners are jointly employed by the university and the practice base, while some are paid entirely by their practice-based employer. In addition, clinical lecturers who are part of the Health Education England/National Institute for Health Research clinical lectureship programme split their time equally between clinical practice and research.

Academics, teacher-practitioners, and teaching fellows normally deliver pharmacy lectures, but you might also have special lectures and classes taken by visitors, pharmacy technicians, nurses, doctors, other industry experts, or university academics from outside of your school of pharmacy. Practical classes, although led by academics, can run with the help of doctoral students, other research staff, or laboratory technicians. Not everyone who teaches on a pharmacy course will have a pharmacy degree or pharmacy registration, but your university will have a sufficient number of pharmacists to make sure that your course is relevant and up to date. The highest number of pharmacists is likely to be found in the 'pharmacy practice' or a similarly named group in your school of pharmacy. The non-pharmacist academics are likely to be laboratory scientists by background, but some schools also have social scientists, statisticians, and health economists on their staff.

The final category of staff which you should know about is your personal tutor, normally someone at lecturer level or a higher grade who is chosen to take on the responsibility of supporting you and a small number of other students throughout your time at university. Your personal tutor is likely to play a crucial role in your studies and we would advise you to build a good working relationship with them from the very start—they are the person most likely to be on your side should things go wrong and, in any case, to provide you with a reference for future job applications. Please also see the section subheaded 'Building a good working relationship with your personal tutor' later in this chapter.

Gaining access to academic staff

Your first year at university is likely to involve you in a steep learning curve. One of the experiences you might need to prepare for is the apparent inaccessibility of lecturers and other staff compared with the availability of teachers within the pre-university school setting. Pharmacy courses can admit anything from 50 to > 200 students in any one year; one of the complications arising from this is that lecturers will not have time to see instantly everyone who experiences a problem or has a question individually. For most students, this is a very different experience to school, where teachers are somehow always available to answer questions. It is worth bearing in mind that although you might not be able to see a particular lecturer quickly, there will be someone from your school of pharmacy available (e.g. your tutor) or from your university's student support services, whom you can contact instead.

At university, most academics will offer consultations by appointment or will advertise a weekly availability through 'office hours' (e.g. Tuesday afternoons). But, of course, part-time staff and visiting lecturers who are not based at the university can be less accessible. Added to this, your course might be offered across multiple campuses, which can create additional accessibility barriers. Finally, depending on when you contact someone, you might be in competition with many other students who simply got in the queue before you.

Not getting access to lecturers and other staff can create a feeling of isolation and detachment, with some students feeling anonymous and even experiencing a sense of loss for the friendlier teacher relationships they had at school. In the past, large pharmacy class sizes and sharing lectures with students from other courses, especially in the first year, could create super-sized lectures delivered to upwards of 400 students. Although these are rare with fully integrated pharmacy courses, the larger lectures, too, can produce an unwelcome lack of intimacy for some as they struggle to make new friends.

Of course not all lecturers will appear aloof and detached and, as we mentioned above, most schools of pharmacy will also have staff that, by virtue of having a teaching focus, should be more accessible to you as a student. In fact, some would argue that the vast majority of academics are extremely supportive of students and enthusiastically support them and that universities go to a lot of trouble to make sure that you have access to tutors and know how to contact them. Tutors and academics have phone numbers and email addresses which appear on their university homepage, so you can communicate with them during the working week by other means, even if arranging a face-to-face meeting is difficult. In addition, please note that universities differ quite substantially from each other so the descriptions we have given here are not entirely universal. Some universities, for example, operate an 'open-door' policy where students requesting a meeting are seen very quickly.

If you are reading this and are worried about what lies ahead (or, indeed, you can already identify with what we describe here), be assured there are steps you can take to personalize your learning experience—to make things feel like they are working for you at an individual level. To do this, you have to learn to take responsibility for your learning. The term that we will be referring to, 'personalization', is all about making your course a 'customized' experience that is flexible to your requirements and thus caters to your needs. This might sound daunting but the guidance we have outlined in a separate section in this chapter entitled 'Personalize your university learning and succeed in your studies' should be easy to understand and perform. A great deal can be said for believing in one's own ability to influence the university experience for the better. Before that section, though, we will examine another concept that sometimes takes new students by surprise, that of academic expectations.

Ways in which academics communicate information

A complaint commonly made by students about university learning is that they do not at first understand the way in which academics communicate with them. Students can find the whole process difficult to grasp and understand and this can be a major problem. Clearly, if your lecturer does not adequately explain what they expect from you, then you will not be able to meet their expectations. Academics sometimes state in their defence that students do not listen to the instructions given to them, but this is not necessarily true. The more universal experience is that some academics still use passive ways of communicating with students and until you as a student get to learn about these (or you encounter academics who adopt more active communication strategies) it can be very difficult to come by some of the essential information that you need, especially in the essential first few weeks.

For example, criteria and instructions are sometimes written in a range of course material and students are expected to find information from these sources, at times without any cues. Without knowing that this information exists and needs to be accessed, students are left not knowing what is expected of them.

This problem is, to some extent, compounded by virtual learning environments (e.g. Blackboard) because academics post information and take it for granted that students will find and read the postings in good time. At the same time, there can be very little face-to-face explanation of some crucial material from academics. Far from being 'spoon-fed' information, students can feel that they do not actually know the criteria for marked pieces of work, which can cause frustration and disappointment. A further twist is that marked coursework can lack a clear explanation as to why a certain (lower than expected) mark was given. Students often think this amounts to poor or insufficient feedback. As we mentioned earlier, do not despair as there are ways of taking things into your hands. The latter part of this chapter contains ample advice on how you can help yourself to a better learning experience. Before that, we are going to look at another important concept which is the global aims of the pharmacy degree.

Appreciating the aims of a pharmacy degree

Another important difference you will encounter at university is the language that is used to describe everything from teaching to assessment to feedback. As well as the general university language, for example, reference to programme specifications, module/subject/unit descriptions, course outlines, handbooks and booklets, assessment schedules, reading lists, virtual learning environments, summative assessment, and so on, there is also specific language associated with pharmacy education. So our aim is to outline the aims of the pharmacy degree, describe some of how pharmacy is taught and assessed, and in the process familiarize you with some of the stock phrases and 'norms' that you will encounter throughout your course.

Most UK universities currently deliver an accredited 4-year MPharm degree that will prepare you for a 52-week pre-registration training year. The pre-registration training is normally provided by a practice base (e.g. community or hospital pharmacy) after which you are required to pass a registration assessment conducted by the General Pharmaceutical Council (GPhC). A minority of universities offer a 5-year intercalated degree that includes within it the pre-registration training. In the future, it is possible that the 5-year intercalated degrees will become the norm.

Whichever format is followed, your course will be made up of individual components, which can be called modules, subjects, units, and so on. Each component will have a certain number of university credits attached to it; credits are simply a way of showing how individual components of a degree fit together to make a viable programme. A typical undergraduate year will involve studying 120 credits so, overall, for a 4-year MPharm degree you will need to study 480 credits. It is worth pointing out that what you study in each year of your degree becomes progressively more complex as you proceed through your degree from the first through to the final year. Each module (or subject or unit) will normally have a description (or handbook or guide) (e.g. module description) that details the number of credits, content, aims, learning outcomes, syllabus, assessment strategy, and timetable for that particular component. A separate document for your course (e.g. course guide or course handbook) will detail the general structure of your degree course, which components make up your degree, whether they are compulsory or optional, and so on. An important point to address is the aim of a pharmacy course.

The GPhC sets out very clear guidance about what pharmacy courses should achieve, expressed as a set of learning outcomes, which are quite extensive. The GPhC is the independent regulator for pharmacists, pharmacy technicians, and pharmacy premises in Great Britain. One of its main functions is to approve qualifications for pharmacists and pharmacy technicians and accredit education and training providers. The essence of the GPhC learning outcomes is that students should study and train safely and effectively, ethically and lawfully, and they should understand and apply principles, methods, and knowledge relating to biomedical and pharmaceutical sciences, psychology, social science, and population and improvement sciences. So, as well as learning about how medicines work, the aim of a pharmacy course is to teach you about how *people* work and how work systems operate.

In the process of learning the curriculum, you are also expected to gain a range of core and transferable skills to inform your future practice. These skills include professionalism, critical appraisal and the ability to interpret and interrogate scientific and clinical data, problem solving, clinical decision-making, accurate record-keeping, reflective practice, effective communication, the ability to analyse and use numerical data, and pharmaceutical numeracy, as well as literature searching and research skills. We would add to that list skills of empathy. Pharmacy degrees also aim to prepare students for career-long learning; as a pharmacist you would need to engage in continuing professional development to keep your knowledge and skills up to date. Your university will no doubt use some form of personal development planning to help you ultimately take full responsibility for your learning and personal and career development in a structured and supported way. The aim of this book is to help you get ahead by learning how to learn these essential skills.

If you wanted to be the perfect university student, you might consider whether there is such a thing as the ideal pharmacy student. A range of behavioural features associated with professionalism in pharmacy students can be mapped according to four dimensions of inter-personal and social skills, responsibility, communication skills, and appearance, the detail of which is listed in Box 1.2. As a pharmacy student in the UK today you will also be bound by the GPhC's code of conduct for pharmacy students, which outlines the attitudes and values expected of you.

The GPhC's current code of conduct is a student-friendly document based on the same seven principles that you will adhere to as a registered pharmacist—although note that these were being revised at the time of publication. These are:

1. Make patients your first concern.
2. Use your professional judgement in the interests of patients and the public.
3. Show respect for others.
4. Encourage patients and the public to participate in decisions about their care.
5. Develop your professional knowledge and competence.
6. Be honest and trustworthy.
7. Take responsibility for your working practices.

 Box 1.2   The range of behaviours associated with professionalism in pharmacy students

Interpersonal/social skills

Diplomatic

Empathetic

Respectful

Non-judgemental

Cooperative

Accepts and applies constructive criticism

Puts others' needs above his/her own

Demonstrates accountability

Behaves in an ethical manner

Maintains confidentiality

Responsibility

Uses time efficiently

Self-directed in undertaking tasks

Punctual

Reliable and dependable

Follows through with responsibilities

Produces quality work

Demonstrates a desire to exceed expectations

Prioritizes responsibilities effectively

Active learner

Communication skills

Communicates assertively and articulately

Demonstrates confidence

Communicates using appropriate body language

Appearance

Practises personal hygiene

Wears appropriate attire

It is crucial for you to adhere to the student code of conduct, that is, the seven principles outlined above, right from the outset of your course. Pharmacy is a regulated health care profession, and carries both privileges and responsibilities, and as a pharmacy student you have to demonstrate you are able to exercise those privileges and bear those responsibilities. This means that you have to conduct yourself professionally at all times. In fact, the GPhC makes it a requirement for schools of pharmacy to have a 'fitness-to-practise' procedure for pharmacy students and if you do not abide by the code of conduct then you might find yourself subject to those procedures. Students who are found to be in serious breach of the code of conduct might not be allowed to progress with their pharmacy course or to register as a pharmacist with the GPhC in due course.

At the time of going to press the *code of conduct for pharmacy students* was still in operation, but a consultation was taking place to consider further aligning students' code of conduct with that of practising pharmacists. The *code of conduct for pharmacy students* indicates how the pharmacists' principles apply to you as a student, showing what is expected of you. Some are especially relevant to you while at university, while others may be more important during placements or work experience and generally off campus. Ways in which you can apply the code of conduct during your time as a pharmacy student are outlined in Box 1.3. This code of conduct is for students studying on accredited MPharm degrees, Overseas Pharmacists' Assessment Programmes, and foundation degrees in pharmacy. It is important, therefore, for you to also have an understanding of the sorts of things that could be seen as potentially breaching the code of conduct (see Box 1.4).

 Box 1.3 Examples of how you can apply the code of conduct for pharmacy students during your course

Principle 1: Make patients your first concern. *For example, maximize your learning on campus and make sure that you put the health and safety of patients first when off campus (e.g. when you are on a placement visit).*

Principle 2: Use your professional judgement in the interests of patients and the public. *For example, challenge others' judgement if their decisions compromise patient safety (e.g. in patient-facing environments).*

Principle 3: Show respect for others. *For example, treat all your fellow students with the same level of respect and don't let any personal biases or prejudices affect your behaviour towards others (e.g. in group work).*

Principle 4: Encourage patients and the public to participate in decisions about their care. *For example, learn how to listen to people and how to involve patients and carers in joint decisions and patient-centred care.*

Principle 5: Develop your professional knowledge and competence. *For example, take responsibility for your learning, attending classes, reflecting on feedback, and making rational and informed choices.*

Principle 6: Be honest and trustworthy. *For example, don't copy other students' work, make sure you collect experimental data accurately, and abide by the rules and regulations of your university.*

Principle 7: Take responsibility for your working practices. *For example, attend classes and dress and behave appropriately; if you are ill and this is likely to affect your work, then tell your university.*

> **Box 1.4** Examples of where a concern might be raised under the code of conduct
>
> Receiving a criminal conviction, caution, reprimand, or penalty notice of disorder or equivalent, relating to certain types of offences.
>
> Behaving in an irresponsible manner due to alcohol misuse.
>
> Using illegal drugs, and novel psychoactive substances ('legal highs').
>
> Aggressive, violent, or threatening behaviour.
>
> Persistent inappropriate or unprofessional attitude or behaviour.
>
> Cheating or plagiarizing.
>
> Dishonesty or fraud, including dishonesty outside the professional role.
>
> Health concerns and lack of insight or management of these concerns.

Your pharmacy course will be designed to instil the skills, values, and behaviours that you will need as a pharmacist, using a range of teaching and assessment methods. Although the rest of this book is devoted to helping you learn from these activities and meet assessment expectations, it is worth outlining here the range of methods that you might encounter through your course.

During the course of your undergraduate degree, you will undoubtedly experience lectures, laboratory classes, pharmacy practice classes, workshops, tutorials, seminars, problem-based learning (PBL) cases, team-based learning, and perhaps computer-assisted learning. You might learn with other professionals (inter-professional learning) and you might interact with patients within the university setting. Certainly you will be required to undergo practice placements—these are periods spent in a pharmacy practice location, for example in community or hospital pharmacies. Additionally, you will conduct a research project or write a major dissertation. Throughout your course, you can expect to be assessed through different activities that might include essays, practical reports, dispensing tests, law and ethics exams, posters and oral presentations, *viva voce* oral exams, reflective writing, PBL assessment, objective structured clinical examinations, patient history taking, and end-of-year or end-of-module/subject examinations. We will cover most, if not all, of these topics throughout the rest of this book.

Personalize your university learning and succeed in your studies

So far, this chapter has outlined some of the challenges students face when starting university, as well as informing you generally about the academics involved in teaching pharmacy and their aims and expectations. Our aim was not to daunt you but to prepare you so that you can have a realistic expectation of university life from the outset. We mentioned earlier that far from being powerless, there are many recognized ways in which you can help yourself to a personalized learning experience; this section includes advice on how you can take matters into your own hands to tailor-make your pharmacy course.

Building a good working relationship with your personal tutor

The top advice is for you to develop a good working relationship with everyone from your personal tutor, to placement tutors, to academic staff, and other students. This might sound obvious, but you will be surprised at the mileage you can get out of good relationships with the people around you, especially if things go wrong or you need extra help and advice. For some people, building good relationships comes easier than for others, so if you need to focus your efforts on one relationship, it should be the one with your personal tutor. Work at establishing the relationship with your tutor right from the very start because what you put in is what you will get out.

In the first semester, introduce yourself to your tutor and share with them your worries and insecurities. Attend all your personal tutor meetings and make a real effort to prepare for each meeting by charting your progress and writing down unanswered questions. This will allow you to engage fully with your tutor, create a good impression, and, of course, to obtain the study advice that you actually need. Do not be afraid to arrange additional tutor meetings if needed. Continue sharing your thoughts and plans with your personal tutor and turn up to meetings enthusiastic and with your own agenda. Most personal tutors have experienced a range of students, or at the very least have themselves been through the university process so they are likely to be empathetic and helpful when you need them to be. Certainly, in the first semester or term, you will have a lot of information thrown your way and the personal tutor can be a good person to untangle the mass of information for you.

If you find that you are just not able to gel with your personal tutor, be clearer about what you want from them. If things do not improve, do not be afraid to contact someone higher up (e.g. a senior tutor) to ask for help. If things have no prospect of improving ask for a different tutor. It might not be possible to change tutors, but it might be worth asking the question at least.

Contacting academics if you need help

Although personal tutors are there to support you in your learning, they will normally direct you to the module leader/convener for specific course-related questions. Remember, if you have a question to ask about a piece of coursework that is going to be marked, ask it early on and do not leave it until the deadline for submitting the work is approaching. As well as having to face competition from other students for the academic's time, the person you want to see might simply not be around when you need them—they might be attending a conference, for example, or be giving an invited lecture. You could try emailing your question to them instead. Of course, you should check the virtual learning environment for the information you are seeking before emailing academics. Please remember that if you send an email to anyone working at the university make doubly sure that you phrase it without the use of slang language and use correct spelling and grammar. You are so much more likely to receive a helpful reply promptly if you send a specific and well-thought-through email in the first place. Please also remember to use your university email address and not your personal one as university staff are only permitted to respond to emails from university accounts, owing to confidentiality rules (see Boxes 1.5 and 1.6).

This has been sent from a private email account and there is no way of verifying who the sender is—the email account name appears as unprofessional

 Box 1.5 Types of emails you should not be sending to academics and why

Unclear what conversation the student is referring to and which dissertation. No apology for apparently taking leave during teaching and an expectation that they can take a class test when it suits them, outside of the scheduled time.

Example 1:

From: bornapharmacist1990@yahoo.com
To: a.brand@university.ac.uk

I told you during the last session for our dissertation that I am not going to be available because I was going to croatia. i was not able to postpone my travelling so i wanna do the class test when i come back.

First name

Sent from my Samsung Galaxy smartphone.

Unclear who the student is, what course they are studying and what year of the programme they have reached.

Example 2:

From: readyforparty@aol.com
To: a.brand @university.ac.uk

Sorry, mustve missed that email I'm in building on Mon 10-11, so can meet him in the foyer after

Sent from aol on Android.

Same comments as above—this student is replying to an email sent to them so some of the missing information is possibly covered in the previous exchange. Nonetheless, the name is missing, they are replying using a private email and they have not taken the time to correct spelling, grammar, punctuation.

Lecturers can be under many different pressures, which you would not necessarily know about (or appreciate), but you can help get a response by thinking carefully about what exactly you are having difficulty with and what advice you are seeking. Of course, make sure that you read all the module/subject material before emailing a lecturer so that you are not asking a question that is already answered in standard course material. Also remember not to make the mistake of addressing academics simply as 'Miss' or 'Mrs', for example. Address them by their title and surname (e.g. Dr Smith) or by their first name if they tell you that they prefer this. But remember it is your right as a student to ask for help, so rather than feeling intimidated by what we have written, we hope this will empower you to contact academics appropriately when needed. Academics that do not do so at first will, with time, show their kindness and empathy, especially as they get to know you and your year-group.

Box **1.6**   Examples of correct ways to write emails to academics

Example 1:

From: [name.surname]@university.ac.uk
To: a.brand@university.ac.uk

Dear Dr Brand

I am [first and second names] currently in year [...] of [name of programme]. You may recall I spoke with you briefly in the workshop [name of workshop] on [date of session]. I am sorry that due to urgent family-related reasons, I have to travel to Croatia next Monday, therefore missing the class test as part of [name of module/subject/unit]. I will be away for a week. Please could you let me know if there is any possibility that I could take the test on my return, a week on Monday? I would be very grateful for your help and advice.

Best wishes [or similar, e.g. kind regards]

[First and second names], [Programme of study], [Year of study]

Example 2:

From: [name.surname]@university.ac.uk
To: a.brand@university.ac.uk

Dear Dr Brand

Many thanks for your email and my apologies for not replying earlier. I can confirm that I will be available to meet with [name of person being referred to in correspondence] on Monday [date] at 11am after my lectures. I would like to suggest meeting in the foyer of the [name of building].

Best wishes [or similar, e.g. kind regards]

[First and second names], [Programme of study], [Year of study]

Making use of student networks

So far we have talked about relationships with your personal tutor and other academics. Most universities also offer mechanisms for meeting other students and gaining useful insights from them. If you are offered these, make use of any student guides during pre-arrival visits or during induction and other possible occasions. These students will have gone through the same process you are about to experience and so they can give you the inside perspective on your university and the pharmacy department. After that, if your university offers a 'buddy system', take full advantage of it.

A student buddy is someone who is assigned to help you—and most students feel comfortable asking him/her questions which they simply would not ask an academic. Your 'buddy' might have even completed the modules/subjects you are taking so they could potentially help answer some general study-related questions. For example, they might advise you on which books are worth purchasing and which are accessible from your university library's online resources. Be careful, however, to not ask for copies of work as you do not want to run the risk of plagiarizing—the reproduction of material that was originally written by someone else without appropriate referencing or permission. Plagiarism is covered in more detail in later chapters, starting with Chapter 4, 'Finding and understanding information', and then in Chapter 5, 'Writing good essays'.

Another way in which you can help yourself is to join the local pharmacy students' association. That way, you can get to meet students in other years of the course and obtain their perspective and advice. Join the national British Pharmaceutical Students' Association (BPSA) and attend their conferences and study days. Although the conferences may not cover subjects directly assessed by your course, the extracurricular activities are bound to give you a more rounded curriculum vitae (CV) and material to put on future job applications. Better still, nominate yourself to be a student representative, either on local committees or for the BPSA.

Taking responsibility for arranging placements and looking into other opportunities

Depending on which university you are attending, look into opportunities to take part in study exchanges abroad. Erasmus is the European Commission's flagship educational programme for university students; if your university offers it, the programme can be a great way of expanding your experience and gaining an edge over others. Take responsibility for your future career by applying for summer placements early on and taking advantage of any careers fairs and careers advice. Make your own network of pharmacy contacts by forming positive relationships with people you come across in the pharmacy workplace. You could also ask around about summer research projects and apply for a position if something is available. A number of academics offer 6-week-long funded research projects, supported by external or internal institutions, and these are normally offered competitively to students in the middle years of their studies (second- and third-year students).

Taking your learning into your own hands

Try to become independent in your learning. Access electronic material such as virtual learning environments regularly, and read all material relating to your modules/subjects. As we mentioned earlier, it is a significant mistake to think anyone other than you holds the responsibility for your learning. For each module/subject you are studying, access the written module/subject description and other material as soon as you can and read the aims (what they hope to teach you), the learning outcomes (what you should have learnt by the end), the other skills you will gain, the timetable, the schedule and methods of learning, the assessment requirements, and, most importantly, the deadlines. Attend all the classes and take responsibility for preparing notes and meeting deadlines—and do not be afraid to provide feedback to lecturers when possible. Download exam papers in good time and practise answering questions in advance of the exam revision period. If your university does not offer past exam papers then enquire about sample exam questions and sample exam papers.

Exercise any choice that you are given, be it in electing project or dissertation titles, or communicating your placement preferences. You probably will not experience many instances where a clear choice is offered so take every opportunity you are given. Make sure you provide a clear rationale for your preference if you have the chance to sway a decision your way (e.g. to be awarded the project you want).

Scrutinize the university webpages—especially the library pages—to see what is on offer. These will normally host a wealth of information about your course, who to contact if things go wrong, study advice, academic rules, and so much more. These webpages will also normally store past exam papers if your university makes such a provision.

Remember to undertake personal development planning (PDP). Use the PDP system offered by your university to identify your needs and chart your progress. This information can inform your discussions with your personal tutor. As part of this process, recognize your learning style—this is covered in more detail in Chapter 2, entitled 'Learning from lectures'.

Of course, the ultimate piece of advice you have already taken in accessing this book—we strongly advise you to learn how to learn effectively. Work through the chapters of this book either sequentially or as the interest takes you, but make sure that you apply our advice and take responsibility for your own learning.

 Key points

- Pharmacy is a full-time university course that requires a full-time commitment.
- The shift to university learning can be challenging for a number of reasons and so it becomes important to prepare yourself for the transition to becoming a pharmacy student.
- At university, you are expected to become an independent learner, which means taking on full responsibility for your daily activities and longer-term plans.
- Familiarize yourself with the material that describes your course, including the programme specification, course outlines, handbooks, assessment schedules, and so on.
- Your course will aim to equip you with a range of core and transferable skills, including professionalism, reflective practice, and communication skills.
- Pharmacy students should adhere to the principles and code of conduct that pharmacists abide by.
- A whole range of staff can be involved in teaching on a pharmacy degree course, some with a teaching focus, some with a research focus, and some with both.
- It is essential for you to develop a good working relationship with all of the university staff and educators you come into contact with, especially your personal tutor.
- Make sure that you address university staff appropriately, especially if writing to them using email.
- Make the best use of any student networks available to you.
- Try and arrange your own pharmacy work experience in addition to what your university offers.
- Engage in personal development opportunities and exercise any choice you are given, for example in terms of project selection.

Further reading and references

British Pharmaceutical Students' Association: http://www.bpsa.co.uk/

Continuing professional development in pharmacy: https://www.pharmacyregulation.org/education/continuing-professional-development

Erasmus Programme: http://www.erasmusprogramme.com/

The Royal Pharmaceutical Society: http://www.rpharms.com/home/home.asp

Student code of conduct: https://www.pharmacyregulation.org/education/pharmacist/student-code-conduct

Subject benchmark for pharmacy: http://www.qaa.ac.uk/en/Publications/Documents/Subject-benchmark-statement—Pharmacy.pdf

2

Learning from lectures

 ## Overview

This chapter is all about lectures. We are going to cover ways in which you can maximize your learning from lectures, including different ways of making lecture notes and engaging with a variety of lecture styles. To do that, we will first describe different lecture formats and styles that academics use to deliver their lectures. People learn differently, so we will also use this chapter to help you identify your individual learning style so that you can work in a way that best suits you.

Almost all universities now provide a copy of the lecture slides or handouts electronically through virtual learning spaces either in advance, or certainly after the formal lecture has been delivered. Some even provide an accompanying video (vodcast) or audio-recording (podcast) alongside the slides, or blend it all into an online lecture (e-learning). Our strongest advice is for you to attend all scheduled lectures when they are given live. Pharmacy students who attend lectures do so because they want to make their own notes, they believe academics provide more information during the lecture or highlight particularly important knowledge, they find the material hard otherwise, or they are simply interested in the course.

There is a lot you can learn by sitting among your peers and actively engaging with the material being delivered. For example, you can learn by watching the professional behaviours of your pharmacy lecturers and you can demonstrate your own professionalism and enthusiasm by interacting appropriately with other students and the lecturer. The most important skills to put into practice in a lecture, however, are effective listening, participation, and note-taking. This chapter focuses especially on these essential skills.

 ## Learning outcomes

You should be able to demonstrate knowledge and understanding of the following after working through this chapter:

- how recognition of learning styles can help with learning;
- how to learn from lectures through preparation, engagement, and reflection.

What are lectures?

For the purpose of this chapter we are going to make a distinction between standard scheduled lectures and e-learning lectures. We will explain what each of these generally involves.

A standard scheduled lecture features an academic, normally standing at the front of a lecture theatre, giving you and others in the audience a presentation live and in person, using a set of slides or other audio-visual material. Although the standard software for producing lecture slides has been Microsoft PowerPoint® for a number of years, there are other alternatives, such as Prezi, that are gaining popularity. In addition, the lecturer might use video as part of the lecture, they may bring in some pharmacy-related medicines and devices for you to pass around and examine, or they might use an audience-response system (think *Who Wants to be a Millionaire!*) to get you to interact with them. The lecturer might ask you to turn to another student next to you to brainstorm a topic, or they might ask lots of questions and expect you and others to shape actively the content of the lecture. Whatever format the lecturer uses, standard scheduled lectures normally last about 1 hour and are based around an academic interacting with you in a physical lecture space on the university campus.

Electronic lectures (e-lectures), however, are delivered over virtual-learning environments (VLEs) such as Blackboard and Moodle. Such e-lectures are not the specific focus of this chapter. However, most of the tips and ideas in this chapter can be applied just as well to e-lectures and other online learning.

Lectures are very useful because the academic will bring together material that is not available in any one source to teach you new knowledge and skills. For example, the lecturer might highlight similarities and differences between different classes of medicines (proton pump inhibitors vs histamine H_2 receptor antagonists). Proton pump inhibitors are drugs such as omeprazole that stop the secretion of stomach acids by blocking what is known in short-hand as 'the proton pump' (the hydrogen–potassium adenosine triphosphatase enzyme system of the gastric parietal cell). Histamine H_2 receptor antagonists, however, are drugs such as ranitidine that block histamine H_2 receptors in order to reduce the amount of stomach acids. Your lecturer might therefore highlight some of the similarities by discussing the general uses of these medicines and then highlight the differences by detailing the specific indications, cautions, and side effects.

Alternatively, your lecturer might present a patient case and ask you to think about which class of medicine would be most suitable to them based on other knowledge. Of course, no matter how good the academic is in preparing and delivering their lecture, the learning part relies on you. Whether you learn in the lecture theatre or afterwards through further work and other reading is all down to you. You should think of the lecture as an introductory way of stimulating you to do further private study based on the information, ideas, concepts, methods, and so on, that were presented to you. At no point should you think of a lecture as the only information you need to study for your module or subject. Students who learn only lecture contents rarely do well in exams. Instead, you should undertake additional reading using the recommended textbooks and study material. One way of getting the most out of lectures, and other learning activities, is to recognize your own learning style and act to increase your potential, which is the focus of the next section.

Recognizing your learning style

We all learn differently. To reflect these differences, Honey and Mumford categorized people (students and adult learners) as being one of four types: 'activists', 'reflectors', 'theorists',

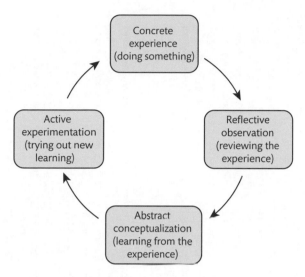

Figure 2.1 David Kolb's experiential learning cycle.

and 'pragmatists'. Honey and Mumford also developed the 'learning-style questionnaire', which can be used to identify your preferred style of learning. This work was based largely on David Kolb's 'experiential learning cycle', shown in Figure 2.1. For Kolb, learning starts with a concrete experience, which is followed by reflection, conceptualization, and, finally, active experimentation, and so the cycle continues.

There are many other ways of defining learning styles. For example, there is the VARK questionnaire, which focuses on identifying people's preferences for learning as visual, aural, read/write, kinaesthetic (practical/physical), and proposing relevant learning strategies (see Table 2.1).

The main focus of this section is to outline the four different learning styles according to Honey and Mumford, and to summarize their usefulness. This does not mean that this is the most valid model. In fact, some academics and researchers believe that none of us can or should be 'typed' rigidly into these or any other categories, and that we might form specific learning styles through habit, or might use different approaches depending on what we are learning and the situation we are in. With this caution in mind, the remaining paragraphs of this section focus on defining the four learning styles identified by Honey and Mumford, with relevant recommendations and examples for each. These four learning styles are summarized in Table 2.2.

Activists

If you are an *activist* then you will generally like attending lectures and other classes so that you can interact and meet other students. You enjoy new experiences and challenges, prefer not to work alone, and you might get bored easily. You might like brainstorming exercises, group discussions, taking part in quizzes and competitions, role-play activities, as well as problem-solving tasks. If you recognize this style in yourself then the standard advice for

Table 2.1 The VARK guide according to preferred learning styles

Learning style	Description	Recommendations for intake of information	Recommendations for learning	Recommendations for performing well in tests
Visual	Prefers symbols and different formats, fonts, and colours to emphasize important points	Access pictures, videos, posters, slides, flowcharts, underlining, different colours, highlighters, books with pictures and diagrams, graphs, symbols, and white space (blank areas)	Turn notes into learning packages by using techniques listed in previous column; reconstructing images or spatial arrangements in different ways; redrawing pages from memory; replacing words with symbols/initials; looking at revision notes	Draw; use diagrams, write exam answers, recall pictures made in revision notes, turn visual images back into words
Aural	Prefers information that is spoken or heard and uses questioning to learn	Attend classes, discussions, tutorials; discuss topics with other students and academics; explain ideas to others; use a tape recorder; remember the interesting anecdotes (stories, jokes); describe a lecture to someone else; leave spaces in notes for later recall	Turn notes into learning packages by expanding on notes by talking with others and collecting notes from other sources; putting summarized notes onto tapes and listening to them; asking others to hear your understanding; reading your notes aloud; explaining your notes to others	Practise writing answers to old exam questions beforehand. Imagine talking with the examiner; listen to your voices and write them down; spend time recalling ideas; speak your answers inside your head
Read/write	Prefers learning by reading and writing	Use lists, headings, dictionaries, glossaries, definitions, handouts, textbooks, readings, notes, essays, manuals	Turn notes into learning packages by writing out the words repeatedly; reading notes repeatedly; rewriting ideas into other words; organizing diagrams/graphs into statements; turning actions/charts/reactions/flow diagrams into words	Write lists; write exam answers; write paragraphs, beginnings and endings; arrange words into hierarchies and points
Kinaesthetic	Prefers using experiences and 'real' things (including pictures/on screen)	Use all your senses (sight, touch, taste, smell, hearing); attend lab classes, placement trips/tours; take a hands-on approach; use trial and error; collect examples; use products, samples; use formulae, past papers	Turn notes into learning packages by using examples in your summary notes, and case studies to help with abstract concepts; talking about your notes with another person; using pictures/photographs; recalling real events	Write practice answers and paragraphs beforehand; role play the exam situation in your own space

Adapted from VARK learn website (http://vark-learn.com/).

Table 2.2 Summary of learning tips according to the Honey and Mumford learning styles

Learning style	Description	Helpful tips for learning
Activist	Prefers interacting with others, quizzes, competitions, role plays and new experiences; prefers not to work alone	Study for short periods; check through your work; review feedback; supplement your notes soon after lectures; make time to work alone
Reflector	Prefers working at a slower pace to others, thinking things over, receiving feedback, observing others	Make clear timetables for coursework and assignments; keep pace with lectures; access e-learning; avoid over-reflection
Theorist	Prefers working logically, analysing problems, managing time, examining theories, factual knowledge, statistics	Avoid over-perfecting coursework and assignments; approach innovative teaching with open mind; see value of applying your learning
Pragmatist	Prefers seeing practical application of theories and trying out activities, and applying learning in practice	Engage in non-preferred activities including discussions, debates, reflection; learn theories, arguments and science of pharmacy

enhancing your learning experience is for you to study for shorter periods (rather than plan a whole day of revision), make sure you check through your work (e.g. essays and assignments) before submitting it, and review feedback when provided. You will probably enjoy interacting with other students and the lecturer in a scheduled lecture.

The most important advice relating to lectures is for you to make sure that you review your lecture notes soon after making them and that you follow up on the lecture effectively. This is because as an activist you will probably busy yourself with lots of interactive, group commitments, and yet it is also important for you to engage in more solitary activities such as supplementing lectures. With e-learning lectures, make sure that you make a schedule and work through the material in short, defined periods so that the work does not pile up.

 Case study   Example of *activist* learning style

Sanjeev was a popular and proactive pharmacy student. He often volunteered answers in lectures, helped out during university admissions activities and was a student representative or president on a number of groups and committees. He was also very popular with academics, who thought him a very intelligent and responsive student and often approached him for feedback about the course and consulted with him on changes and improvements planned for the future. All of this activity came at a cost: Sanjeev struggled to keep up with his lecture notes.

He saw a library notice about an exam study skills workshop and thought it worth attending, even though exams were soon approaching. One of the most important points that Sanjeev took away was guidance on how to prioritize his time so that he focused on his studies over and above all his other activities. The workshop inspired Sanjeev to download a smartphone application (app) that allowed him not only to timetable his revision, but which also then interacted with Sanjeev by sending reminders and asking for progress on timetabled activities.

Sanjeev went ahead and used the app; although his exam results were not as high as he had hoped that year, he used the method in subsequent years to keep a focus on his studies. Sanjeev is now a successful pharmacy manager and leads an active and satisfying personal and professional life.

Reflectors

If you are a *reflector* then you will generally like working at a slower pace to others, preferring to think things over before rushing to a conclusion. You might like one-to-one informal discussions, receiving feedback from other people, completing questionnaires, or other activities focusing on your learning style and personality, observing other people, and being coached to reflect on your development and future plans, as well as conducting interviews and taking time out from formal class activities. You probably will not volunteer to answer questions in interactive lectures, choosing, instead, to stay anonymous.

If you recognize this style in yourself then the standard advice is for you to make clear timetables for coursework and assignments that allow you to break down tasks and manage your work effectively. This is because as a reflector, you will probably busy yourself with thinking over the detail of what you are learning, and yet it is also important for you to actually get on with activities and keep to deadlines. Of course, you then also have to make sure you are monitoring your progress and sticking to your timetable, or changing it as needed. The most important advice relating to lectures is for you to make sure that you keep pace with presentations and do not ponder over the detail of what is being said too much or you will soon fall behind with your note-making. You might find that you enjoy e-learning more than standard lecture classes.

 Case study   Example of *reflector* learning style

Jo was a considerate and kind pharmacy student. She never responded to invitations to share views or answer questions publicly in lectures. Although some found her to be shy and somewhat reserved, to those who knew her well Jo was an extremely sympathetic and thoughtful friend. Jo had noted that she often left interactive practical classes that focused, for example, on 'responding to symptoms', feeling dissatisfied with her own performance. She found it difficult to give precise, straightforward advice, but she was not sure how she could improve on this in light of the vast array of information to filter and choose from.

A lecture on decision-making triggered Jo to reflect on her decision-making style and so she asked a friend for feedback on her decision-making through a role-play scenario. Jo's friend thought that, although very empathetic, Jo erred too much on the side of caution, and gave indecisive advice and unfocused answers. Jo reflected on this feedback and devised a flow chart to help her in future consultations. The flow chart involved her making notes actively during a consultation, obliging her to differentiate between minor symptoms and more serious symptoms. Based on this approach, Jo then found she could give clearer, more decisive advice, having made a decision about the potential severity of the symptoms earlier on. Jo is now a very successful formulary pharmacist at a large teaching hospital.

Theorists

If you are a *theorist* then you will generally work logically, in an organized and efficient way. You will enjoy analysing and solving problems, and managing your time. It is likely that you will like learning about models and theories, as well as statistical and factual knowledge, and hearing other people's stories, quotes, and background information as part of your studies. The standard advice is to make sure that you do not spend too much time perfecting course-work and assignments before submitting them. The most important advice relating to lectures is for you to keep an open mind because you might not take well to more innovative lecture styles, preferring the traditional noninteractive lecture type, for example. You might not see the point of case studies, preferring instead to focus on theory and factual knowledge. This is because as a theorist, you will probably busy yourself with learning facts and theories, and yet it is also important for you to learn how to apply the theories in a pragmatic course such as pharmacy. Make sure that you attend all lectures, even though some might involve a format you are not used to.

 Case study   Example of *theorist* learning style

Paul was an academically talented student. He achieved particularly high exam marks before starting his pharmacy degree, and saw himself as someone who would sail through and obtain a first-class degree before pursuing a career in research. Indeed, Paul's academic performance at university was impressive and he obtained high marks in all his written assignments in his first year. But Paul found it quite hard to apply his learning in some of the classes and workshops that involved interacting with others.

When he performed badly in an assessed exercise focusing on emotional intelligence, the workshop leader recommended that Paul stops and thinks about why he does not perform as well in face-to-face situations and to spend some time addressing this issue. When Paul reflected on this, he thought that although he clearly understood the theory of emotional intelligence, when faced with a pretend patient in practical classes, he found it impossible to know how to apply the theory. Having identified this weakness, Paul worked to his strengths and searched on the Internet to find some useful example videos which bridged the gap between theory and application.

Paul is now completing a PhD in pharmacy and using his understanding of emotional intelligence when he interacts with his supervisor and other postgraduate students.

Pragmatists

If you are a *pragmatist* then you will enjoy seeing the practical application of theories, for example through case studies and patient examples. You will certainly enjoy being given the chance to try activities for yourself, for example taking someone's blood pressure or noting their medication history. You will probably like being given problem-solving tasks, as well as being given time to think about how you can best apply your learning in practice. The standard advice is to make sure that you try and engage in all available activities, even those that do not at first appeal to you (e.g. theoretical discussions, debates, and reflective activities). The most important advice relating to lectures is for you to remember that understanding theories and different arguments are the bedrock of pharmacy so make sure that you learn these, as well as the practical elements of the course. This is because as a pragmatist, you will probably busy yourself with applying the learning, and yet it is also important for you to actually understand the underpinning science of pharmacy.

 Case study   Example of *pragmatist* learning style

Suzy was seen as an excellent pharmacy student. She sailed through her entrance interview, having shown plenty of commitment to pharmacy through work experience and placements. She did very well in her pharmacy practice classes and showed excellent communication skills. Although her course took an integrated approach, Suzy recognized a particular problem with some of the theory and factual knowledge that was being taught. For example, she found it very difficult to understand and commit to memory what she was taught on renal physiology and the structure and function of the kidney. She mentioned this to the lecturer who showed Suzy an online resource where she could interact with a visual display of the kidney and its parts, and different substances in the blood as they went through a nephron.

Suzy learnt from this experience and later followed up topics she could not understand by searching for other online, interactive lessons where she could try concepts out for herself. Suzy is now employed as a competent community pharmacist and helps patients understand how to take their medicines through her excellent communication skills.

If you are interested in finding out your preferred learning style then there are ample online tools available to help you do that.

Before we conclude this section on learning styles, we want to say that, in our opinion, the best approach is, in fact, not to typecast yourself as a particular type of learner. Instead, think of your learning style as an indicator of how you normally learn in different settings, with scope for trying new approaches and recognizing what else might also work for you. Some people refer to this as a learning cycle that involves not only engaging with a learning activity, but also reviewing and learning from the activity and planning for the next learning activity, through strategically stopping and thinking at particular points on your course (akin to Kolb's model of experiential learning explained earlier in this section). You might find that your particular pharmacy course has put mechanisms in place to enable you to do this in a structured way. In any case, Chapter 12, 'Continuing professional development', expands on this notion of the learning cycle in the context of reflection and personal development. For now, we will return to the subject of the lecture and, specifically, how to prepare for lectures.

Preparing for lectures

Most people think that if you do some preparation *before* the lecture, then you will learn more from the lecture itself. There is more than a grain of truth in this and so universities are using innovative ways to help students prepare for lectures. For example, some academics define difficult concepts and terminology before a lecture, some ask students to contemplate answers to specific questions, while others assign pre-lecture reading and related activities to encourage students to engage with the material in advance of the lecture. Some are even using podcasts and vodcasts so the pre-lecture material feels personal and engaging in a similar manner to the lecture itself.

It is great news if your university lecturers put thought and effort into providing you with pre-lecture instructions in this way, especially if you then make use of what is available. Our strongest advice, then, would be for you to engage actively with the pre-lecture material if you can. However, if you do not receive this sort of structure, you can still prepare for lectures—and this section provides you with some helpful tips on what steps you can take. Remember, the onus should be on you to prepare yourself at university. So although it is a bonus if your lecturer does provide pre-lecture guidance, do not rely on other people to do the work for you!

Firstly, find out if copies of the lecture slides or handouts are going to be made available on your course's VLE before the lecture takes place. If not, then look at the title of the lecture and see if you can find more information about what might be covered in the lecture by cross-referencing against the course or module booklet. This resource usually describes the overall aims and learning outcomes of the course or module that the lecture forms a part of. If all you find is a lecture outline then have a look in the recommended textbooks or on relevant websites to get a feel for the topic, especially if it is new to you.

You might also want to think about how the lecture might add to existing lectures and the course or module as a whole. Do not go overboard—you do not need to do more than about 30 minutes of preparation before a lecture, but getting a feel for what might be covered will help you think about what you might gain from the lecture and any questions that you might want answered through the lecture.

If the lecture slides or handouts are, in fact, made available on the VLE beforehand, then we would advise that you print and read these in advance. Some people prefer to view slides electronically and even take notes in lectures electronically. This is fine as long as you learn effectively using electronic material. The point we are making is that you should access and read the slides or other lecture material before the lecture if these are made available. Nothing will replace the experience of hearing the academic speak to the words that you will read online or on paper, so do not be fooled into thinking that the slides are an effective substitute for attending the actual lecture. You will learn why, below.

During the lecture

In a lecture, it is likely that you will spend the first 15–20 minutes listening attentively (or you will, at least, have every intention of doing so). But, if you are like most other people, after that time you will become less interested in what the lecturer is saying and more interested in your other thoughts. This is especially true of specific types of learners such as activists, as described earlier in the section 'Recognizing your learning style'. Some lecturers recognize this and will introduce a new activity or topic at around the 20-minute point. Some will introduce gaps in lecture handouts that require you to keep up with the material to fill in the gaps. Others, however, will continue to work through their material in a consistent manner from beginning to end. Your job throughout is to try and listen and understand what the lecturer is saying, ideally making notes as you do so. By making notes, you will process and understand the lecture.

Some people would argue that students should make a conscious effort to sit near the front of the lecture theatre to improve their engagement with the lecturer and the content being presented. Certainly, if you make effective notes, you will not only help your concentration, but also feel much more that you are learning, there and then, from the lecture. Actively making notes will help you retain much more of the information from a lecture than just passively sitting and listening.

But how do you listen effectively and take notes at the same time? We are not suggesting that you should write down *everything* that the academic is saying. There is little point in doing that if you have a full copy of the lecture slides in front of you. (We will describe what you should and should not include later in this section.) Remember, also, that while it might be useful to make an audio recording of the lecture (if permitted) or use a podcast if routinely made available, these are no substitute for actively listening and learning from the lecture experience. So do not be fooled into a false sense of security through the knowledge that you have a copy of what is being said: no one ever has time to go through every single audio-recording of a lecture for note-making later on. Indeed, although useful to some people for revision purposes, listening back to lectures can also be very time-consuming compared with revising from lecture notes.

Listening and taking part

Your lecturer might begin by telling you the learning objectives and the importance of the lecture, as well as outlining the lecture content. Listen out for these and try to use them as headings for your notes. For example, your lecturer might say 'The point of this lecture is to help you understand how each anticoagulant works, as well as the potential advantages and disadvantages of each medication'. (This is the learning objective.) Then they might state 'The National Patient Safety Agency put out a Patient Safety Alert relating to anticoagulants, listing actions that will make anticoagulant therapy safer in 2010' (which flags the importance), be- fore moving on to say 'today we will cover warfarin, its action, interactions, and side-effects, as well as...' (at which point they are describing the lecture content).

The body of the lecture itself should be organized into *chunks* of knowledge; you can try to anticipate these by looking at the lecture content in advance. The lecturer might use other clues relating to the structure of the lecture, which can also help you with organizing your notes, including 'Moving on to another class of anticoagulant...', or 'These three classes of drugs are the mainstay of anticoagulant therapy...'.

As you sit and listen, try and think actively about what the lecturer is saying: how does it fit with what you already know; does it throw up more questions; do you agree with what they are saying; does it all make sense; are they repeating points or emphasizing specific points? In this way, you will be using the learning style of reflective learners, if you are not one already. Your mind might wander to other topics, in which case bring your thoughts back to what is being said. The use of patient cases by the lecturer might well appeal to pragmatists, but if you tend to be more of a theorist when it comes to learning, try and grab the opportunity being presented to you. Remember that case studies are a great way of demonstrating the applica- tion of theories and knowledge to real-life situations.

Finally, look out for non-verbal messages. These might be difficult to interpret at first, but tone of voice, pauses, and repeats can indicate the importance and significance of topics being discussed. Towards the end of the lecture you should definitely listen out for the im- portant take-home messages. What are the main points and concepts you are being asked to remember? You might be in a very interactive lecture, so you might be asked to respond to the lecturer's questions, discuss something with a partner, or complete a quiz or vote on different options instead of listening on your own. We have already talked about the fact that only some types of learners enjoy this type of activity. If you are more of a reflective learner, try making full use of the opportunity—you might surprise yourself with the results. Finally, if you have a question and are given the chance to ask it, then please take the chance to do so.

Writing effective lecture notes

Some people believe that effective note-making is about occasionally writing down important points during a lecture, as and when they arise, while others believe that making good lecture notes involves transcribing everything as you hear it. Clearly, neither of these approaches can result in a coherent stand-alone set of notes for your later use. If you only note down important points, you might miss the overall context; if you try to write everything down it can become impossible to keep up with the lecture and you can end up with incomplete notes. In addition, trying to write everything down will make it a passive, automatic activity that will stop you from actively listening and learning from the lecture.

Certainly, if you have a copy of the lecture slides or handouts in front of you, it can become tempting simply to underline certain words, copy down additional diagrams, or fill in gaps in lecture slides, but active note-making involves far more than that. If you can print a copy of the slides or the handout beforehand, use this as a framework for your own note-making. Just make sure that you print the slides in a way that leaves plenty of space for annotations and notes. Remember that making effective lecture notes is crucial for exam revision so it is important to get this right if you can.

Our first advice then is to make sure that whatever you write down is *in your own words* instead of verbatim statements by the lecturer. Paraphrasing what is being said will make you *bring your own meaning* to the material. For example, imagine that your lecture is on anticoagulants and your lecturer says the following: 'Remember, warfarin comes in four strengths in the UK. It is important that the patient understands this. Usually they will be issued with at least three strengths and it is vital that they or their carers can work out how to translate a dose in mg into the correct number of tablets of the correct colours'. Imagine also that the lecture slides being presented show the different-coloured tablets with the following text: '4 strengths available in UK: 0.5 mg—white; 1 mg—brown; 3 mg—blue; 5 mg—pink', separated by bullet points. If you make linear notes, we would expect your notes to read something along the lines of: 'Warfarin tablets are colour-coded and each colour indicates a different strength. The highest strength tablet is pink (5 mg), followed by blue (3 mg), brown (1 mg), and white (0.5 mg). It's our job to help patients and carers work out which dose to take'. This is what we mean by paraphrasing what the lecturer is saying. You can see that the process of summarizing and rewording what you hear will make you interpret what is being said. This kind of active engagement is great for enhancing your learning.

Listen out for and write down words and phrases that your lecturer keeps repeating; if you have already made a note of these, underline or circle the important concepts. Write down additional examples and any anecdotes the lecturer provides. Also, make sure you note down key words that summarize the overall message, for example 'platelet activation', 'prothrombin time', and 'International Normalized Ratio (INR) testing'. Active note-making will also involve you in noting down any questions that come to mind or points that you want to follow up later. For example, you might write 'Look for warfarin packets next time in the dispensing class' or 'Ask to see a copy of the anticoagulant booklet' or 'Comparison with new oral anticoagulants (NOACs)?'.

We would also encourage you to develop a system of abbreviations: this will also help you make effective lecture notes more speedily. As you progress on your pharmacy course, you will be taught a whole range of pharmaceutical and medical abbreviations—try and use these in your lecture notes as much as possible. Some Latin abbreviations are listed in Table 2.3 and some medical abbreviations in Table 2.4. There are also a number of short-hand symbols and abbreviations that students tend to use, some of which are listed in Tables 2.5 and 2.6.

Table 2.3 Some examples of Latin pharmaceutical abbreviations

Abbreviation	Meaning
a.c.	*ante cibum* (before food)
b.d.	*bis die* (twice daily)
o.d.	*omni die* (every day)
o.m.	*omni mane* (every morning)
o.n.	*omni nocte* (every night)
p.c.	*post cibum* (after food)
p.r.n.	*pro re nata* (when required)
q.d.s.	*quarter die sumendum* (to be taken four times daily)
q.q.h.	*quarta quaque hora* (every 4 hours)
Stat	*immediately*
t.d.s.	*terdie sumendum* (to be taken three times daily)
t.i.d.	*ter in die* (three times daily)

Adapted from *British National Formulary*, latest edition.

Table 2.4 Examples of medical or other abbreviations

Abbreviation	Meaning
Rx	Prescription
Tx	Treatment
Sx	Symptoms
Dx	Diagnosis
IV	Intravenous
IM	Intramuscular
NKDA	No known drug allergy
Caps	Capsules
Tabs	Tablets
N&V	Nausea and vomiting
Ung	Ointment
Aq/H_2O	Water
Disp	Dispense
MDI	Metered dose inhaler
D.O.B.	Date of birth

Table 2.5 Examples of short-hand symbols

Symbol	Meaning
%	Percentage
&	And
~	Approximately
+	Plus
=	Equals
<	Less than
>	More than
?	Why
×	Times
±	More or less
♀	Female
♂	Male
∴	Therefore
c	With

Table 2.6 Examples of short-hand abbreviations

Abbreviation	Meaning
approx.	Approximately
c.f.	Compared with
e.g.	For example
etc.	Et cetera (and so on)
excl.	Excluding
i.e.	That is
incl.	Including
ltd	Limited
max.	Maximum
min.	Minimum
N.B.	Note
no.	Number
v.	Very
vs	Against

Note-taking methods: linear notes versus visual diagrams

Some people learn by making linear notes during lectures. This involves starting at the top of the page and working straight down; writing short sentences, key points, and abbreviations; and using headings, subheadings, bullet points, numbering, and underlining to organize the text, provide emphasis, and group ideas into specific chunks. If this works for you, then try to leave

Box 2.1   Example of linear notes

What we mean by health behaviours

There are three types of related behaviours:

- Health behaviours—preventing disease
    - e.g. good diet
- Illness behaviours—seeking a remedy
    - e.g. going to the pharmacist
- Sick-role behaviour—aiming to get better
    - e.g. taking medication.

plenty of space in between your writing to enable you to go back and make additions later on. One of the disadvantages of linear notes is that it can be difficult to see how each section fits in the overall theme of the lecture unless you are particularly careful. This can be tackled later—for example, by numbering the major headings and adding a summary list of all the major topics. See Box 2.1 for an example of linear notes from a lecture on patient behaviours.

A different method of note-making involves using diagrams, maps, and drawings to provide more structure and better cross-referencing between different concepts. Some people use specific types of drawings called mind maps or spider diagrams. These types of notes are very helpful to people who prefer to learn visually and are a great way of showing how the different subtopics fit into a whole. The idea with mind maps is that you would start by writing the main heading in the centre of the page; you would then devote one out-going branch to each subheading and so on with other smaller headings and concepts.

You can either use small mind maps for different subtopics during a lecture or make one large mind map to cover everything. Of course, we are not suggesting that you take a large A3 sheet of paper to your lecture room for producing the large mind maps. Instead, if you make small mind maps in the lecture, then you might want to think about writing up your notes afterwards in a way that includes all of the concepts in one diagram.

Mind maps are great for showing all the relevant concepts and their interrelationships at a glance and can be very helpful for revision purposes. Some people get very creative, using different-coloured pens for different ideas, adding diagrams and drawings, as well as symbols and other details to help with learning and recall. See Figure 2.2 for an example of a mind map.

A hybrid of linear notes and the mind map is the flow diagram, which is particularly helpful for showing processes or other concepts that involve movements or associations (see Figure 2.3).

Of course, quite a number of students also now use electronic devices for recording their lecture notes, either during or after the lecture, in addition to the traditional note-making method of using pen and paper. These technology-based strategies can range from tapping words into a laptop using software such as Microsoft Word and PowerPoint to drawing on digital notebooks. Alternatively, digital pens give you the best of both worlds: they allow you to still write on paper, while having the added advantage of converting your writing to a digital page. If your budget allows, do experiment to see which method you prefer.

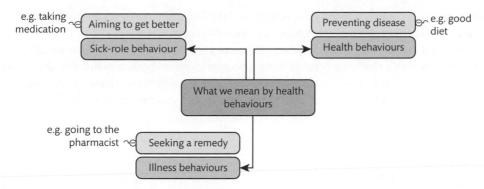

Figure 2.2 Example of a mind map.

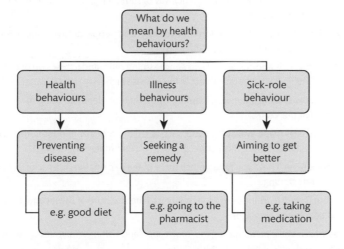

Figure 2.3 Example of a flow diagram.

Actively learning from lectures afterwards

A fantastic way of preparing for your revision is to visit your lectures notes soon after the lecture so that you can begin to commit the learning to your long-term memory stores. Go over the material to check for unclear or ambiguous areas. Read your notes and think about what you have learnt from the lecture. What were the main points? Why was the lecture important? Can you start applying your learning in the course? If so, in which workshops and practical classes? Do parts of your notes need to be supplemented with further reading and research? What questions does the lecture raise in your mind?

Make a plan for what you need to do to as a result of reading your notes. You might want to contact the lecturer or you might use your initiative and look on the VLE for additional information first. Some people find it helpful to rewrite their notes after a lecture, to help make the information easier to read and understand at a later date. Some prefer instead to just annotate their notes and add in lines and drawings to clarify relationships and help link concepts better. If you remember examples that the lecturer gave or responses from other students, you could also make a note about these afterwards.

The key is to make sure that you do actually make the time to revisit your lecture notes; this can be particularly challenging for *activists*, who prefer new experiences instead. Once you are happy with your lecture notes, do not simply file them away in an organized way: you will need to think about how often to revisit your notes so that you can reinforce the knowledge and work on further memorizing that lecture content.

 Key points

- Lectures are useful because the academic will bring together material that is not available in any one source, to introduce you to new knowledge and skills.
- You should think of the lecture as an introductory way of stimulating you to do further private study based on what was presented to you.
- People learn differently, and Honey and Mumford categorized people as being one of four types, namely activists, reflectors, theorists, or pragmatists.
- The VARK questionnaire is another way of assessing learning style, and focuses on people's preferences for learning as visual, aural, read/write, or kinaesthetic.
- Recommendations exist for helping each learning style, whether identified using the Honey and Mumford method or the VARK.
- If pre-lecture material is made available to you, such as lecture slides or handouts, then you should work through this material before the lecture, printing relevant material if needed.
- Actively making notes will help you retain much more of the information from a lecture than just passively sitting and listening.
- Look or listen out for the learning aims, clues relating to the structure of the lecture, non-verbal messages, and take-home messages.
- Good lecture notes involve paraphrasing the information and writing it in your own words rather than verbatim according to what the lecturer states.
- A range of short-hand symbols and abbreviations can help make the process of note-making faster.
- You can experiment with your note-making by writing them in a linear fashion, using flow diagrams or by drawing mind maps on paper or by using an electronic device to test which style you prefer.
- Make sure that you make the time to revisit your lecture notes either to rewrite them or annotate them to help make the information easier to read and understand at a later date.

 Further reading and references

Honey P, Mumford, A. The Manual of Learning Styles. 3rd ed. Maidenhead: Peter Honey; 1992.

VARK Learn Limited. The VARK questionnaire [online]. Available from: http://vark-learn.com/the-vark-questionnaire/ [Accessed 21 July 2015].

Westrick SC, Helms KL, McDonough SK, Breland ML. Factors Influencing Pharmacy Students' Attendance Decisions in Large Lectures. Am J Pharm Educ. 2009 Aug 28;73(5):83.

Learning in the laboratory

 ## Overview

This chapter focuses on laboratory practical classes that relate to the science subjects underpinning pharmacy. The science of pharmacy spans the processes of drug development and usage, encompassing a range of topics:

- the understanding of cellular and molecular pathways and sites of drug action;
- the discovery of therapeutic agents and toxicological and pharmacological experiments;
- the extraction/synthesis, analysis and assay of drug compounds;
- the formulation, manufacturing, and packaging of drugs;
- trials in humans, marketing and usage by patients, all the way through to post-marketing surveillance.

The science of pharmacy can even encompass the withdrawal of a medicinal product from the market.

Viewed in this way, the science of pharmacy is not limited purely to laboratory research but does stem from it. Therefore, laboratory-based practical classes are often used as a fundamental component of pharmacy courses and we will explore this important topic in this chapter. Your practical classes can centre on separate or integrated drug development or related processes to help you to learn the scientific method and its application to pharmacy.

We are going to cover the many ways in which you can maximize your learning from laboratory classes. To do that, we will first describe what we mean by science, scientific prediction, and exploration. We will then cover health and safety, as this is a crucial component of laboratory working. Finally, we will concentrate on communication of science by considering practical reports and scientific papers. We will not cover the fundamentals of statistics at all because there are other books available that teach this important topic in depth.

 ## Learning outcomes

You should be able to demonstrate knowledge and understanding of the following after working through this chapter:

- health and safety concerns in the laboratory;
- the scientific method of enquiry and the basics of an experiment;
- what information to put into an experimental report.

What are practical classes?

For the purpose of this chapter we are going to make a distinction between real ('wet') laboratory classes and 'virtual' laboratories carried out using e-learning tools. We will first explain what each of these generally involves.

A real practical class involves you attending a laboratory to engage physically with an experiment in real time, either individually or in groups. Therefore, you might reasonably be asked to learn how to handle chemicals, biological compounds, equipment, and apparatus, and use the fixtures and fittings (e.g. bench, fume cupboard, etc.) in a manner that is in line with rules on health and safety. As well as general laboratory skills, you will be likely to learn a range of very specific practical skills involving, for example, conducting acid–base experiments, handling cultured cells, running enzyme kinetic studies, using skin to measure drug release, running chromatography assays, and so on.

But practical classes are not limited to the laboratory. Nowadays, a range of computer software is used in order to mimic real ('wet') laboratory experimentation; such 'virtual' labs could also form an integral part of your course. These virtual packages allow you to design and simulate real-life experiments without having to conduct the work in a physical environment.

Of course, there are advantages and disadvantages to both methods and you might find that your school of pharmacy uses one method in preference to the other, or a combination of the two. Our focus in this chapter is on the physical laboratory experience, although most of the tips and ideas in this chapter can be applied just as well to e-learning packages.

Health and safety considerations in laboratory-based classes

Practical classes in a pharmacy course are likely to involve you in a wide range of activities. To study safely it is important that you follow the rules set out by the class supervisors. Having gained entry onto a pharmacy course, it is likely that you will have already observed certain laboratory health and safety rules and practices in your prior learning—for example, wearing lab coats and goggles, and not consuming food and drink while in the lab.

What we want to highlight here is that it is not just the responsibility of your university (or place of work, e.g. on an industrial placement) to provide you with safe working conditions (e.g. specifying the rules, conducting risk assessments, providing the right safety equipment). It is also your responsibility to follow the rules and report any issues to a safety officer. You might even encounter an accident in the lab, and again it is your responsibility to report this and follow appropriate procedures or advice. All laboratory classes are equipped with a first-aid box, and names of trained first-aiders should be clearly displayed alongside other emergency information, such as what to do in a fire.

In addition to fire and accidents associated with equipment and apparatus, specific harm can arise from mishandling chemicals or biological compounds in the laboratory, with exposure possible through inhalation, ingestion, absorption by the skin, or splashes in the eye. For example, sensitizing chemicals can cause skin allergies and respiratory reactions, carcinogenic compounds can cause or be suspected of causing cancer, mutagenic compounds are implicated in gene mutations, and teratogenic compounds can cause malformations in an embryo or fetus. In addition, biological substances (e.g. material containing viruses and bacteria) can potentially cause infections, and other health problems. A number of pictograms are used in order to alert people to the possibility of harm, and some of these are shown in Table 3.1. It is your responsibility to read the cautions and handle all potentially hazardous substances with appropriate care.

In addition, Box 3.1 provides a basic list of laboratory safety rules. In preparation for each class, read and follow the specific precautions given to you for minimizing risks to health and safety from hazards associated with the chemicals and techniques being used. All practical classes should be accompanied by safety instructions; you should refer to and adhere to the guidelines issued by your institution. You must bring in a laboratory coat if this is a requirement of your course. It goes without saying that you must maintain a high standard of discipline and practice in the laboratory by accurately following the correct schedule of work and working cleanly and tidily.

The scientific method

The very nature of pharmacy courses ensures one certainty: it will be impossible to predict and list the full range of practical classes and experiments that you will encounter. This is because you are likely to measure and collect data relating to a range of concepts (see Table 3.2). Rather than repeat guidance that will accompany your practical classes, we will cover some universal ideas, starting with the concept of the scientific method.

Whichever way your pharmacy experimental classes are run, they will share one very distinct feature: they will be based on the scientific method, the idea that knowledge is based on what can be recorded through the senses. In other words, what you see is what you get (and what you should believe).

Although this might sound obvious, as you progress through the course you will learn that there are other ways of working that do not rely so much on observation and recording but more on interpretation and guesswork. For example, capturing patients' personal feelings and views about their health and illness can rely on a completely different framework to the laboratory sciences. But our focus here is on the scientific method.

The basis of the scientific method is the idea that information can be gathered and then analysed in a pre-planned, methodical, and even-handed way by skilled scientists. The 'facts' then derived from such analysis are backed up with firm evidence, rather than simply being based on one person's conjecture. The ultimate outcome of scientific work is to generate new knowledge that might one day become accepted scientific law.

To do their work, scientists take great care to focus their experiments and laboratory work on a limited number of 'things' (known as variables) to be studied in the lab. In other words, scientists simplify experiments so that they can answer one question at a time. To make sure that their results are not contaminated by other effects or variables, scientists also work in a controlled laboratory environment, using very clear procedures and working carefully and precisely every time.

Think of a baker in a kitchen—the work of the scientist and the baker are not too different in many respects. Both must have a limited list of ingredients, a careful procedure to work to, and a safe and clean environment in which to operate. Imagine the outcome if the baker decided to change the listed ingredients for other ones, worked in no particular order, and

Table 3.1 Examples of hazard symbols that specify potential danger

Pictogram	Description
	Explosive, self reactive, organic peroxide
	Respiratory sensitizer, mutagen, carcinogen, reproductive toxicity, systemic target organ toxicity, aspiration hazard
	Corrosive (causes severe skin burns and eye damage), serious eye damage
	Harmful skin irritation, serious eye irritation
	Acute toxicity, very toxic (fatal), toxic, etc.
	Gases under pressure
	Flammable gases, flammable liquids, flammable solids, flammable aerosols, organic peroxides, self-reactive, pyrophoric, self-heating, contact with water emits flammable gas
	Harmful to the environment
	Oxidizing gases, oxidizing liquids, oxidizing solids
	Biological hazard

Adapted from the UK Health & Safety Executive website, www.hse.gov.uk.

Box 3.1   Basic safety rules relating to laboratory settings

Safety in the laboratory

- Familiarize yourself with emergency procedures.
- Read the statements relating to control of substances hazardous to health (COSHH).
- Always wear a buttoned-up (fastened) laboratory coat.
- Wear goggles or safety glasses where advised.
- Wear gloves when you are handling chemicals, sharp objects, and other materials hazardous to health.
- Avoid inhaling powders and wear a mask as appropriate.
- Use the fume cupboard, extractor fan, or other containment facilities appropriately, when instructed to do so.
- Do not eat, drink, smoke, chew gum, use a mobile phone, apply make-up, or engage in any other activity likely to compromise your safety while in the lab.
- Do not handle equipment or materials using your mouth—e.g. never pipette by mouth or lick labels.
- Place all broken glass in a suitable broken-glass bin and place all needles and syringes in a suitable sharps bin.
- Wash your hands and remove gloves by using the correct technique before touching communal surfaces (e.g. computer keyboards, telephones).
- Do not undertake any experiments other than those specified by the class leaders.
- Do not leave any potentially hazardous procedures unattended.
- Dispose of all waste correctly using the specified procedure.

cooked outside on a barbecue—they would end up with a very different product to the one they intended to produce.

Rather than making original scientific discoveries, most of your laboratory classes will be based on existing procedures. Therefore, very much like the baker (or the baker's apprentice) you will be expected to follow a carefully written set of instructions to explore the science for yourself. But, unlike the baker's apprentice who wants to end up with a perfect bake at the end of their efforts, your desired outcome will be a set of measurements (or 'results' as they are formally known).

Table 3.2   Examples of different types of data you might generate in your laboratory classes

Muscle physiology	Dissolution	Cell count	Concentration
Enzyme kinetics	Absorbance	Age	Volume
Blood pressure	Chromatography	Mass	Microscopy
Time	Temperature	Heart rate	Partition coefficient
Capacity	pH	Viscosity	Sugar levels

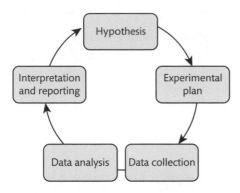

Figure 3.1 The research process starts with a hypothesis, which leads to a careful plan of experimentation, according to which the experiment is run and data are measured and analysed before being interpreted and reported.

In an experiment, therefore, you can expect to focus on a limited number of variables, observing and measuring their behaviour while accounting for or avoiding interference from other unwanted variables. Data in the laboratory always take a defined, measurable, and factual form.

The different stages of an experiment

A number of stages underlie the scientific method. These include the generation of a hypothesis, experimental design, the carrying out of the experiment and measurement-taking, as well as analysis, interpretation, and reporting (see Figure 3.1). Depending on the nature of your laboratory class, the experiment will be based either on a hypothesis or an established scientific law but will invariably involve measuring responses or reactions.

The hypothesis

A hypothesis is a statement describing the predicted relationship between at least two variables and the idea is that through rigorous and repeated testing, a hypothesis can become scientific law. For example, you might form a hypothesis that the storage of medicines in compliance aids at room temperature will result in significantly greater drug degradation compared with storage in the refrigerator. If you prove the hypothesis to be correct through rigorous testing, then you could recommend that medicines in compliance aids are stored at cooler temperatures.

Of course, experiments do not always work out in predicted ways and hypotheses are sometimes rejected or replaced by new ones. A hypothesis is simply a suggested explanation for a set of measurements that may or may not be supported by the experiment (see Box 3.2). Bear in mind that it is important for a hypothesis to be based on some prior context; this could be prior theory, experience in practice, reports from patients, or previous research. If your laboratory class is based on an established scientific law, as it often will be, then rather than testing a new hypothesis, the practical will have been designed to help you understand one of the fundamental sciences of pharmacy, by enabling you to experience the science for yourself.

Box 3.2 Some general features of a hypothesis

Checklist for a hypothesis

- Is based on theory or previous research findings.
- States a relationship between at least two variables.
- Is a simple and clear statement with no vague terms confusing the relationship.
- Is realistic and testable so that the measurements can actually be made in practice.
- Has the capability of being accepted or refuted; the prediction can be evaluated in terms of 'yes, it occurred' or 'no, it did not occur'.
- Is related to known and available techniques of design, procedure, and statistical analysis.

The experimental variables

A standard experimental practical will almost always require you to measure and compare the relationship between two or more variables, one (or more) of which is known as the independent variable and will be controlled by you, the experimenter. The other variable is the dependent variable and will change as a result of the different conditions of the experiment.

For example, storage temperature is an independent variable—you can control and manipulate it according to your instructions. One of the authors of this textbook has experimented in the past with storing tablets at different temperatures (e.g. standard room temperature and hot summer temperatures), to examine any effect on chemical breakdown of the drug. The quantity of intact drug present in the tablets, when measured using an assay, then becomes the dependent variable—it changes (or is hypothesized to change) as a result of storage temperature.

It is crucial that you choose (or are given) a dependent variable that produces valid and measurable data. Manipulating the independent variable and measuring the resulting changes in the dependent variable allows you to infer the relationship between the two. For example, if we store chloramphenicol eye drops at room temperature rather than in the refrigerator (with temperature being the independent variable), our measurement of drug composition (the dependent variable) will decrease, showing drug degradation. We can then infer a relationship between storage temperature and drug degradation. In fact, chloramphenicol eye drops have to be stored in the refrigerator because a higher temperature does, indeed, accelerate the breakdown of the active drug component.

Take another example: a practical class designed to demonstrate the relationship between simulated lung function and vital capacity (the volume of air that can forcibly be blown out after full inspiration). You can use a spirometer (an instrument for measuring the air capacity of the lungs) in order to measure vital capacity, which would be the dependent variable here. You might then measure your vital capacity under three experimental conditions: normal setting, simulated restrictive disease (by securing a belt around your chest) and simulated obstructive disease (by using an altered mouthpiece that allows only a small flow of air). Lung function then becomes the independent variable in this experiment with three conditions

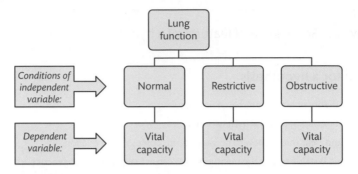

Figure 3.2 Lung experiment example. The independent variable is manipulated to create three experimental conditions (normal, restrictive, and obstructive lung function) and its impact on the dependent variable is then measured (vital capacity readings).

(normal, restrictive, and obstructive function). The hypothesis will describe the relationship between lung function and vital capacity readings (Figure 3.2).

Unwanted variables

There will always be other variables that might also impact on the measured outcomes. As a good experimenter you will recognize these other variables (or be told what they are) and try and control for them, for example by keeping them constant. Can you suggest some other variables that might interfere with the lung experiment described in the previous section and think of ways of controlling for them?

Experiments require the strict control of a number of other conditions with the sole purpose of minimizing interference with the actual experiment to enhance reproducibility. In the example given in the previous secion, if data were being collected from a large number of people for hypothesis testing then you would ensure that all participants have similar normal lung function to start with, can use the belt in exactly the same way (for simulating restrictive lung function), and are provided with identical mouthpieces (for simulating obstructive function). In addition, you might measure participants' gender, age, and health status, to try and control for significant participant differences when making your analysis.

It seems obvious, therefore, to say that once the details of an experiment have been worked out, you must carry out the procedure with the utmost care. Poor experimental technique can introduce many potential biases that could wrongly infer a different relationship between the experimental variables (or even suggest no relationship at all).

Data collection

It is not only the set-up of the experiment that can result in erroneous data, however. You must also make sure that you (or a device) are accurately measuring and recording the experimental outcomes.

The other advice we have, then, is based on the concepts of accuracy and precision (also sometimes referred to as validity and reliability). Accuracy is a measure of how close your

Figure 3.3 Paracetamol weight analogy demonstrating the difference between accuracy and precision. The average weight of tablets is calculated by totalling each weight and dividing by 3 (total number of measurements). The standard deviation is a measure of the spread of weights, with a smaller number indicating higher precision and a larger number, lower precision.

Measuring three tablets carefully on an uncalibrated balance	Measuring three tablets carefully on a calibrated balance	Measuring three tablets carelessly on an uncalibrated balance
610 mg | 612 mg | 614 mg	571 mg | 570 mg | 572 mg	671 mg | 610 mg | 634 mg
Average weight of tablets = 612 mg	Average weight of tablets = 571 mg	Average weight of tablets = 638 mg
(higher than should be, because balance is not calibrated)	*(correct average weight because balance is calibrated)*	*(higher than should be, because balance is not calibrated)*
Standard Deviation = 2	Standard Deviation = 1	Standard Deviation = 30
(small standard deviation because measurements taken carefully)	*(small standard deviation because measurements taken carefully)*	*(large standard deviation because measurements not taken carefully)*
Low accuracy but high precision	*High accuracy and high precision*	*Low accuracy and low precision*

results are to the true value that you should have measured, whereas precision indicates how reproducible your results are.

For example, imagine three students measuring the weight of paracetamol tablets in a pack containing identical tablets, each weighing, on average, 570 mg (accounting for the added tablet excipients). The first student uses the same exact method for each measurement but does not realize that the balance they are using is not correctly calibrated; they consistently measure the weight of each tablet as 40 mg heavier (see Figure 3.3). Their measurements will be precise (each tablet will weigh about the same) but not accurate—as their results will have inadvertently measured the tablets to be heavier than they actually are.

Imagine the second student realizes that there is a fault with the balance, recalibrates it, and then takes careful measurements. Their readings will be both accurate and precise. Finally, imagine the third student neither realizes the fault with the balance nor applies consistent methodology and so ends up with tablets of different weight. They would be neither accurate nor precise.

One way of ensuring accuracy, then, is to calibrate the equipment or machine that you are using for your measurements. Some experiments will require you to produce a calibration curve using standard known concentrations to regulate your findings. We have given an example of a calibration curve in Figure 3.6, later in the text.

Another important point is to check that the machine or equipment that you are using can actually measure in the required range: there is no point using an electronic balance that is only sensitive enough to measure in grams to weigh out milligrams of a substance.

In terms of precision, make sure that you have followed the experimental procedure with care and have controlled for potentially interfering variables (e.g. temperature, humidity, etc.) by keeping environmental conditions constant. You should always take several readings to identify the precision of your measurements. Reproducibility describes the closeness of agreement between sequential measurements, under the same conditions: the same procedure, the same observers, the same instrument used in the same location, with repeated measurements being taken over a short period of time. In one experimental session you would expect your results to be closely reproducible. You will often be told to take three readings and then use the mean of these for your results.

To conduct an experiment properly then, you must work to a specific standard operating procedure in a methodical manner. A standard operating procedure (SOP) is a document containing step-by-step guidance on the correct performance of a task such as your experiment. Your SOP should outline its scope and objectives before providing a list of the materials you require, the equipment that you should use, the procedure that you should follow, the records you should make, as well as safety considerations. By following a SOP you can help ensure that your results are valid and reliable. Box 3.3 provides a summary of a good experiment.

Presenting and interpreting your data

In your experiment you would have created situations in which a limited number of factors would have been manipulated and their effects on the dependent variable measured. The next stages in completing your experiment are to present the data you have gathered in a way that others can readily digest, and then to interpret that data—to determine what that data are actually telling you. Let us focus first on the presentation of data. The mainstay of scientific data collection is the humble results table.

Table of results

As a first step you are likely to be asked to record your measurements directly on paper during the laboratory class or will be using computer printouts or other recordings in order to derive data relating to the dependent variable. Whatever your plans are, it is almost certain

---

 Box 3.3   Crucial elements of a good experiment

Checklist for an experiment

- Hypothesis stating relationship between clearly identified independent and dependent variables.
- Plan for accurate measurement of dependent variable and type of data expected.
- Unwanted variables clearly identified and their impact controlled for.
- Procedure lists equipment, materials, and how to manipulate the independent variable.
- Plan for analysis, including analytical tests.
- Collection and analysis of data according to written procedure.
  - Rejection or acceptance of the hypothesis and interpretation of the findings.
  - Clear and timely reporting including a discussion of the experimental results.

Table 3.3 Example of a raw data collection table

Sample number	Drug concentration (raw measurements)		
	Blister packaging	*Compliance aid I*	*Compliance aid II*
1	113 mg	113 mg	89 mg
2	109 mg	109 mg	88 mg
3	110 mg	110 mg	86 mg
4	120 mg	120 mg	92 mg
...			
Final sample	100 mg	100 mg	101 mg

that your data will be recorded in the form of tables to start with. Table 3.3 shows a raw data table. You would normally be expected to summarize your findings, so as well as the raw table, you would have to use summary tables and potentially graphical ways of presenting your findings.

You will either be told to keep your data in your experimental booklet or you will be at liberty to transfer your data to Microsoft Word to produce printed summary tables. See Table 3.4 as an example of a summary table.

There are many visual ways in which you can present your findings, including the use of pie charts, bar charts, line graphs, and so on. If you are going to create graphs and diagrams, use a software package such as Microsoft Excel to help you.

A pie chart

A pie chart is a circular diagram that will allow you to show how different categories contribute to an overall set of results. For example, you might want to show the estimated amount of protein consumed in a day, according to the type of meal, as noted in a food diary (see Figure 3.4). Although pie charts can be useful when you want to demonstrate that there are visible differences between categories of data, they are not useful when you have many more conditions to represent.

Bar charts

Bar charts are good for demonstrating differences and enabling comparisons between different variables, especially where the independent variables are 'discrete'. Data are said to be discrete when they are related to defined categories of measurement (drug properties, storage containers, meal times) rather than measurements on a scale. For example, Figure 3.5 shows

Table 3.4 An example of a summary results table

	Average drug concentration (mg)		
	Blister pack	*Compliance aid I*	*Compliance aid II*
Room temperature	115.9 mg	111.1 mg	113.9 mg
Raised temperature	113.7 mg	104 mg	113.6 mg

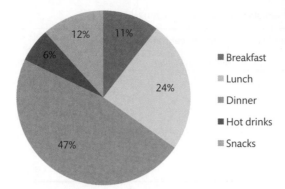

Figure 3.4 Example of a pie chart demonstrating the relative percentage of protein consumed in different meals in one day.

drug concentrations in tablets stored in different containers at two different temperature settings. Here, a rectangular bar proportionately represents the measured drug concentration for each condition and the chart allows two data sets to be shown side-by-side—storage temperature, as well as storage container. In this example, the discrete variable is the storage container (of which there are three discrete categories, shown on the *x*-axis of the bar chart).

Line graphs

You are likely to use line graphs (scatterplots) frequently in your experiments as these are suitable for comparing the relationship between one variable and another, specifically where

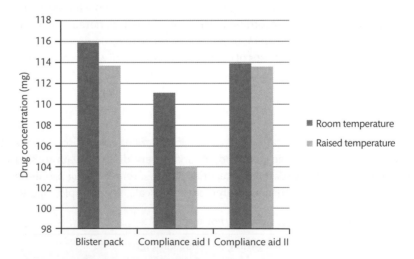

Figure 3.5 Example of a histogram demonstrating the contrast between the drug concentration in different containers and at two different temperatures. Note: the *y*-axis starts at 98 to emphasize the differences, whereas setting this to zero would show the entire data set.

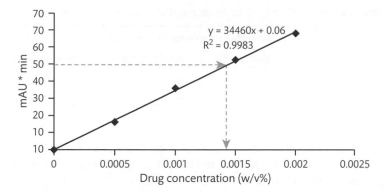

Figure 3.6 Example of a line graph demonstrating the relationship between the area under the peak (from a high-performance liquid chromatography assay) on the y-axis plotted against drug concentration on the x-axis.

both variables are measured on a continuous scale (i.e. neither the independent nor the dependent variables are 'discrete'). Line graphs are used, for example, when creating calibration curves (see Figure 3.6), recording plasma concentration as a function of time, or when demonstrating dose response. Note that drawing a straight line between the points on such a graph makes the assumption that the data *between* the recorded points conforms to the straight-line pattern being drawn.

Figure 3.6 is a calibration curve, a type of line graph in which the response of a measuring device to a series of known concentrations of a substance is plotted. In this example, the drug concentration is plotted along the x-axis, while readings for the area under the peak obtained from a high-performance liquid chromatography (HPLC) machine is plotted along the y-axis. As the drug concentrations increase, the areas under the peak increase in a very linear and proportionate fashion. This particular calibration plot has been obtained by running a series of precise and known drug concentrations through the HPLC machine.

The graph shown in Figure 3.6 demonstrates a very good positive relationship between the drug concentration and measurement through HPLC. This is very useful as it means that the calibration plot can be used to predict the concentration of *unknown* samples based on their own areas under the peak. Imagine running through a sample whose drug concentration you do not know but need to determine through your experimental work. According to Figure 3.6, if you obtain a mAU * min reading of 50 (to denote the area under the peak from the unknown sample you run), you would plot this along the y-axis and then draw a straight line to meet the calibration curve. You would then draw a line straight down to the x-axis to read the drug concentration predicted by the calibration curve.

Interpreting your data

You will be expected to use statistical tools to help communicate and analyse your results. It is outside of the scope of this book to provide a detailed explanation of these statistical tools. However, in broad terms, there are two types of statistical analysis you might need to make use of: *descriptive* and *inferential*.

Table 3.5 The mean and standard deviations (SDs) for an exemplar set of data

	Mean (SD) drug concentration (mg)		
	Blister pack	Compliance aid I	Compliance aid II
Room temperature	115.9 (2.3)	111.1 (2.6)	113.9 (2.1)
Raised temperature	113.7 (2.4)	104 (1.9)	113.6 (2.3)

In simple terms, descriptive statistics provide a general sense of your findings, both by indicating the average value of your data, and by indicating the range of values across which the individual data points are spread.

There are different ways in which averages can be measured, although the most common way is to calculate the mean. The mean of a set of data is calculated by summing up all the scores and dividing the total by the number of scores taken. For example, Table 3.3 lists four measurements of drug concentrations found in blister packaging: 113 mg, 109 mg, 110 mg, and 120 mg. The mean of these four results is found by summing all four values and dividing by the number of values counted (four): (113 + 109 + 110 + 120)/4 = 113 mg.

As well as calculating an average for the values you obtained in your experiments you will also be expected to show some measure of dispersion of the individual data points, such as the *range* or the *standard deviation* (SD).

The range is the difference between the smallest value in your dataset and the largest one and so is calculated by subtracting the smallest value from the largest one. By contrast, the SD tells us how the individual values that make up a dataset vary (or 'deviate') from the mean. For example, Table 3.5 summarizes the mean drug concentrations and SDs for six data sets. (The SDs are the values given in parentheses in each cell.)

The smaller the SD, the more tightly the individual data points were clustered around the mean value calculated. For example, at room temperature, compliance aid I gave a mean drug concentration of 111.1 mg, and a SD of 2.6. This tells us that the individual data points from which the mean was calculated ranged from having a value 2.6 less than the mean to 2.6 greater than the mean. By contrast, at a raised temperature, the same compliance aid gave a mean drug concentration of 104 mg and a SD of 1.9. This tells us that the individual data points ranged from having a value 1.9 less than the mean to a value 1.9 greater than the mean. In other words, the individual data points at the raised temperature were more tightly clustered around the mean (they *deviated less* from the mean) than the data points at room temperature.

You must, where applicable, also analyse your results to determine whether significant differences or relationships exist between individual datasets. This will formally allow you to answer the experimental hypothesis. Such analysis draws on the tools of *inferential statistics*. Inferential statistics use laws of probability to help us make inferences based on information from the experimental data we have gathered.

Imagine that the data you have gathered suggests there is a difference between the experimental groups you are considering. For example, your data may suggest there to be a difference in drug concentrations in the room temperature versus raised-temperature groups, as per the data given in Table 3.5. There is a possibility that such a finding represents a real difference; however, the finding may simply be a product of sampling error: it is *not* a real difference. Inferential statistics give us a way of expressing how confident we can be that this difference is real (or, indeed, false). If we think the difference is real, we say that it is *statistically significant*.

A number of inferential statistics exist; these include *t*-tests, analysis of variance (ANOVA), chi-square (X^2), and regression analysis. The actual inferential statistical test chosen depends on the nature of your data: you can not always use a *t*-test, or a X^2 test, for example. It is likely that your lecturers will already have outlined which statistical test to use and the rationale for doing so, so we will not go into the detail here.

The main point of conducting statistical tests, of course, is to prove or disprove your research hypothesis. You will find that most statistical packages will return descriptive statistics relating to your data; in addition, the statistical test that you use will return a result that will indicate whether there are statistically significant differences between your datasets (e.g. those relating to different test conditions). For example, inferential statistics will calculate a probability value (*p*-value) that shows the chance that your hypothesis is, in fact, true. If the probability value is smaller than at least 0.05, then you might conclude that the difference or relationship is, in fact, statistically significant and you can accept the experimental hypothesis: a probability value of 0.05 tells us that there is a 5% chance (or less) that the difference is due to chance.

Writing your practical report and fuller research papers

You must always write up the results of your laboratory experiment, for two reasons. Firstly, you will probably be required to do this to complete your learning. Secondly, as a scientist, you are obliged to report on your results so that they are accessible to the wider community and can be scrutinized by other scientists. Your report should be clear, accurate, and succinct. It should be written in an objective and dispassionate way using third person, past tense.

A full report will normally be divided into a number of standard sections: title, abstract, introduction, method, results, discussion, references, appendices. Your introduction should contain an aim and objectives section, and the discussion should end with a conclusion section. Typical laboratory classes are unlikely to require full introduction and discussion sections, and you might well be asked instead to focus on the methods, results, and interpretation of the findings.

Students always ask about word counts and the relative proportion of each section in a full report. This very much depends on the specific field within which you are working and the advice you are provided by your lecturers. However, we can provide some general guidance in terms of the content of reports here.

The report title

The title must be precise and concise, communicating what was manipulated and what was measured in your experiment if possible. For example, one of the authors of this book has carried out some experimental work examining the stability of medicines in compliance aids. They gave one of the published papers the following title: 'Quality of medicines stored together in multi-compartment compliance aids'. In hindsight, they could have been more specific and referred to the independent and dependent variables in the title itself: 'The physicochemical stability of tablets stored together at room and higher temperatures in compliance aids'. Still, some people argue that the title of a study should also reveal something about the findings. A more innovative approach would be to say 'Reduction of physical stability on short-term co-storage of tablets in different compliance aids'.

Introduction to your report or paper

If you are asked to write an introduction, you should use this to explain why the experiment was conducted, focusing on the existing literature and providing a clear rationale. For example, you should review previous research and theory relevant to the study. This research could be theories/studies from the textbooks, or from other research and published reports that you have located when conducting a literature search (Chapter 4 focuses on explaining literature searches). Your introduction should show a logical progression, building up to a description of the study. This is your opportunity to use the literature you have found to weave together a convincing argument as to why your study was needed at this point in time. You should start with a more general stance, refining the introduction as you progress. Towards the end, you should state the aims of the study and what you are hoping to achieve.

The introduction usually takes the form of an upside down triangle: it starts wide and becomes increasingly focused until you reach an explanation for your study. For example, for the paper entitled 'Quality of medicines stored together in multi-compartment compliance aids', the author used the introduction to describe what multi-compartment compliance aids are and how they are used in practice. They then explained how against standard stability data, very little data exists on stability in compliance aids, which are devices that offer little protection against physical (light, aid, temperature) and chemical (co-storage with other tablets) conditions. They outlined what was known about formulations that degrade when stored in compliance aids, and explained that the gap in knowledge necessitated further work. They referred to previous experiments in this area and explained how those results still left some unanswered questions. Finally, they outlined a clear research question which flowed naturally from the text that preceded it. They then clearly stated the aim of the study, including the dependent and independent variables.

The method section of your report or paper

The method section should explain very clearly and systematically how you carried out the experiment so as to allow others to repeat the process accurately and be able to mimic your findings. You should explain the study design, the materials, the reagents, and the equipment, as well as the exact procedure. It is conventional to note down batch numbers, serial numbers, expiry dates, and other detail relating to the material and equipment that you used. Going back to the example paper entitled 'Quality of medicines stored together in multi-compartment compliance aids', the author first listed all the products that they had used, where they had sourced them, batch numbers, and expiry dates, as well as descriptions of the compliance aids. They then explained the experimental design, stating:

Three different factors with different levels were applied and their influence on the physicochemical stability of the two generic atenolol tablets evaluated after 4 weeks of storage. The factors investigated were packaging, temperature and co-storage with aspirin tablets. This design meant there were 14 different conditions for each of the two atenolol tablets tested.

They then described, in detail, each physical stability test that they had applied; listing the equipment used as well as the test specifications followed (e.g. The United States Pharmacopoeia 24 (USP 24) specification for dissolution testing). For the HPLC assay (test of chemical stability), they detailed the equipment, conditions, and validation and extraction method. They wrote the method in enough detail that would allow another scientist to copy exactly their experiment to reproduce the same results.

The results section of your report or paper

In the results section, you should detail the data collected, any calculations you performed, the statistical detail and the results of the statistical tests. If your findings are statistically significant, you should very clearly state what the results indicate in relation to your hypothesis, using descriptive statistics to provide context. For example, if we found that there were statistically significant differences in drug concentration between different storage temperatures, we would provide context by stating clearly the actual difference—for example, storage at higher temperatures resulted in lower drug concentrations, indicating higher drug degradation.

Ideally, you should restate the research hypothesis at the beginning of the results section. You should signpost to raw data; for example, if these are in an appendix then you should clearly cross-reference to this material. The results section should provide a summary of the findings, using tables and graphs as described earlier. All tables and graphs should, of course, be clearly labelled. If you used statistics, then you should state which statistical tests were applied, providing a summary of the results of the statistical tests. In addition, you should give a clear statement of the findings in relation to the original research hypothesis. Steer clear of providing any interpretation of the findings; this is purely the domain of the discussion section.

The discussion section

Your discussion should provide a brief summary of the results and relate this to the existing literature and knowledge on the subject. Here, you should interpret the findings. If the results were not as you predicted, then you should explain why this might be the case. Could it have been due to experimental error, or do the results bring into question the original theory? Your discussion should certainly bring the findings back to the theory that you introduced in the introduction. In the latter stages of your course you should also be questioning the validity of your results, by thinking about weaknesses or potential biases in your study, especially if you are conducting novel research (e.g. in your research project). You should also use this space to highlight study limitations and suggest improvements to the study. A good report will also outline the implications of the results and any future work before stating what conclusions can be formed from the findings.

The conclusion should be a final 'sharp' summary paragraph. In the example paper we have been using here, the final conclusion was:

The multi-factorial experimental conditions impacted differently on the physical stability of tablets stored within MCCAs [multi-compartment compliance aids] so conducting relevant research in this area is not realistic and the issue may need to be entrusted to medical device regulators and the professional body for pharmacy.

Other sections of a full report

The abstract is a summary of all the sections of the report; it is usually placed after the title of a full report but can really only be produced properly after the full report has been written. You are very unlikely to be asked to produce an abstract for ordinary laboratory reports. Finally, a full report should be referenced and contain any relevant appendices. Again, you are unlikely to be asked to produce references for short laboratory reports.

Chapter 4, entitled 'Finding and understanding information', provides much more detail about what is normally contained in an abstract, as well as citations and referencing.

The key is to make sure that you follow the instructions you have been given for the particular type of report expected of you. This way, you can learn how to communicate your scientific work using conventional styles, a skill that is essential to working and learning in the laboratory.

 Key points

- The scientific method asserts that knowledge is based on what can be recorded through the senses.
- The science of pharmacy stems from basic laboratory research and laboratory-based practical classes are therefore a fundamental component of pharmacy courses.
- A range of computer software is also used in order to mimic laboratory experimentation in a virtual sense.
- In a physical laboratory you are expected to handle any chemicals, biological compounds, equipment, apparatus, and fixtures and fittings in line with rules on health and safety.
- Familiarize yourself with pictograms that are used to alert people to the possibility of harm and handle all potentially hazardous substances with appropriate care.
- Maintain a high standard of discipline and practice in the laboratory by accurately following the correct schedule of work and working cleanly and tidily.
- In an experiment the aim is to gather information and analyse it in a pre-planned, methodical, and even-handed way by someone with the skills to complete the work.
- You should take great care to focus your experiments and laboratory work on a limited number of 'things' (known as variables) to be studied at once.
- A hypothesis is a statement describing the predicted relationship between at least two variables and should be based on some prior context such as prior theory, experience in practice, reports from patients, or previous research.
- Unwanted variables are those that might also impact on the measured outcomes in an experiment but will be recognized and controlled to stop them from doing so.

- You ensure both accuracy (a measure of how close your results are to the true value that you should have measured) and precision (how reproducible your results are) when completing an experiment.

- Depending on the instructions you have been provided and the context of your work, you can present your findings using tables, pie charts, bar charts, or line graphs.

- You should use an appropriate mix of descriptive and inferential statistics to analyse your data.

- The report of your experiment should be clear, accurate, succinct, and written in an objective and dispassionate way using third person, past tense.

- A full report will normally be divided into a number of standard sections, including title, abstract, introduction, method, results, discussion, references, and appendices.

Further reading and references

Blann A. Data Handling and Analysis (Fundamentals of Biomedical Science). Oxford: Oxford University Press; 2014.

Donyai P. Quality of Medicines Stored Together in Multi-compartment Compliance Aids. J Clin Pharm Ther. 2010;35(5):533–543.

Langley C, Perrie Y. Maths Skills for Pharmacy: Unlocking Pharmaceutical Calculations. Oxford: Oxford University Press; 2015.

Medawar PB. Advice to a Young Scientist. New York: Basic Books; 1981.

World Health Organization. Handbook: Good Laboratory Practice (GLP): quality practices for regulated non-clinical research and development; 2009 [downloadable pdf file]. Available from: http://www.who.int/tdr/publications/documents/glp-handbook.pdf [Accessed 17 October 2016].

4 Finding and understanding information

 Overview

Pharmacists update or check their knowledge frequently by accessing information, so we want to teach you how to find reliable information using different resources right from the first year of your studies. This chapter is about sourcing and understanding the origin of information, a skill that is also essential to writing good essays and research reports during your degree. The skill is also vital for answering pharmacy-related enquiries from patients and other health professionals later in your practice. Box 4.1 provides some examples of activities in your pharmacy degree where finding reliable information is likely to be central to producing good work.

Certainly, the General Pharmaceutical Council would expect pharmacists to know how to access a wide range of pharmacy-related information, including local and national guidelines, to ensure that their practice is based on evidence. Box 4.2 provides some examples of activities in pharmacy practice that necessitate good information handling skills. When you are qualified as a pharmacist you will find that sourcing, managing, and giving information is an essential part of your responsibilities. Any information you give must, of course, be correct, be impartial and up-to-the-minute, and be from a trustworthy source.

In this chapter we will outline the range of literature and sources of information available to you, as well as how you can use scientific databases to find these. We will discuss plagiarism and how to avoid it, which leads us to referencing and referencing styles. Finally, we will show you how to use the Internet credibly. Note that your university's library will no doubt also offer resources and guidance, as well as support sessions on the topics covered in this chapter.

 Learning outcomes

You should be able to demonstrate knowledge and understanding of the following after working through this chapter:

- the different sources of information that are relevant to pharmacy;
- how to search pharmacy-related sources for required information.

Box 4.1   Examples of learning activities that rely on finding good information

- Case-based learning.
- Essay writing.
- Research report.
- Dissertation.
- Problem-based learning.
- Critical review.
- Objective structured clinical examination.
- Practical report.
- Dispensing class.
- Medicines information activity.

 Box 4.2   Types of activities that necessitate finding reliable information in pharmacy practice

- Clinical problem.
- Critical appraisal of literature.
- Preparation of a publishable manuscript.
- Information provision.
- Guideline development.
- Formulary management.
- Drug-use review.
- Audit.
- Preparing bulletins or newsletters.
- Managing entry of new drug into hospital/primary care.
- Managing adverse drug reaction.
- Continuing professional development.

What are the relevant sources of information in pharmacy?

What is the range of information you might need and where might you source these? Pharmacy-relevant information exists in a range of publicly available forms. You might be interested in finding information, for example, in relation to malaria treatment; medical devices; prescribing guidance; chemical safety; health protection; law and ethics; summaries of product characteristics; regulatory matters; professional development; drug misuse; patient information; poisons; medicines information services; toxicity; clinical guidelines; drug mono-graphs; systematic reviews; health-technology assessments; immunization; and injectable medicines. We mention this because there are certain other types of information that are not in the public domain—for example, unpublished laboratory reports or in-house drug-safety reports.

There are two key things to know. Firstly, *what* type of information you need and *where* you can look for it. The different reference sources that contain pharmacy-relevant informa-tion include, for example, websites, science gateways, search engines, books, news reports, journals, databases, blogs, and encyclopaedias. Secondly, you need to know *how* to find the material you need.

As a student you are most likely to use the Internet, rather than reading, say, a printed book. We are not frowning on this, but it is crucial that you know the difference between what to expect from an academic textbook versus information on the Internet or in a scien-tific journal, in terms of validity, as well as scope. Of course, we can now access electronic books through the Internet, so it would be wrong to imply that any information delivered online should be avoided. With this in mind, we are going to categorize information as pri-mary versus secondary rather than making a distinction between electronic and hardcopy paper resources. We will do this by considering what we call the chronology of information.

The chronology of information

A very good way of thinking about information is to consider the timeline along which the knowledge has been produced. Although the Internet gives the impression that there is limit-less information swilling in the universe (or at least online), a lot of this information is, in fact, repeated, or cleverly packaged up in altered formats, for different purposes or audiences. What you find yourself reading on a particular webpage may be several steps removed from the form it took when first written.

Think of the scientific work we referred to in Chapter 3, or any other work that is newly created. This type of information is primary information—it adds new knowledge to what is already known. Other types of information (secondary information) draw on primary in-formation to fill reviews, summaries, books, databases, or compendia. Mostly, these sec-ondary reference sources attempt to repackage primary information for easier access and use. Knowing about the information supply chain, with information going from primary to secondary sources, can help you identify where to look for the type of material you need.

Primary information sources

The term 'primary literature' refers to original studies that are normally published in scientific, academic journals, for example the *British Medical Journal*. It can also include other material such as case reports, case series, committee reports, and opinions, as well as conference proceed-ings, but these other examples do not carry the same credibility as original study publications.

One of the advantages of using a primary reference source to look for information is that you will see the paper in its original form and so will have the opportunity to assess it for

Box 4.3   A brief description of the key individuals involved in bringing about the publication of primary scientific work in peer-reviewed journals

- The *authors* are those who have made fundamental intellectual contributions to a study manuscript and its publication. This can include coming up with the idea and designing the study, obtaining the data, analysing and interpreting the data, drafting the article or revising it critically for important intellectual content, and approving the final version to be published. The authors will normally send their manuscript to a journal for peer review and await a decision about its suitability.

- The *peer reviewers* are experts who are not part of the editorial staff of a journal and who act to assess independently manuscripts submitted to journals for accuracy, originality, and scientific validity, as well as worth and interest to the journal audience.

- The *editor* of a journal is the person responsible for its entire editorial content. Depending on the journal, there may also be associate editors and together the editorial team will make an assessment of the value of a new manuscript before deciding whether it should be subjected to peer review. On receiving the advice of peer reviewers, journal editors hold the final decision on whether a manuscript is to be published or not (and whether changes are needed to the original manuscript).

- Some journals also have an independent *editorial advisory board* composed of experts in the field to establish and ensure editorial policy.

yourself (especially as you gain the skills to do so later in your course). This is a different experience from accessing a book, where information that is written might be the author's interpretation of a published study—denying you the chance to see and assess the original material for yourself.

Original papers are usually the culmination of many years of hard work. Primary research of this sort enters the public domain once the researchers have written and submitted their work to a journal editor. See Box 4.3 for a brief description of key players involved in the production and approval of original primary studies for publication.

Peer review of original studies

Authors of original papers normally create accurate, clear reports of their studies for publication. Once a manuscript is received by a journal, a process known as 'peer review' is used by editors to help decide which manuscripts are suitable for their particular journal. Peer review is considered to be an important part of the scientific process whereby other experts in the field carry out an unbiased, independent, critical assessment of the work (see Figure 4.1).

Peer review also helps authors and editors to improve the quality of reporting, but it can be a time-consuming process. This is because peer reviewers have to make suggestions, and editors have to approve and pass these on to the authors, who then have to send back their changes for further review. A peer-reviewed journal is one that has submitted most of its published research articles for outside review. Therefore, knowing whether a journal upholds peer-review processes is one way of assessing the quality of information you find.

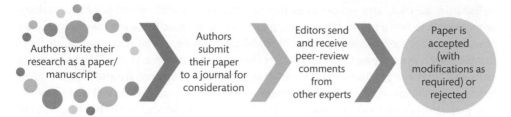

Figure 4.1 A basic schematic of the process from authorship to acceptance of a paper for publication in a peer-reviewed primary reference source.

Journal reporting styles

Most pharmacy-related research publications follow a conventional style, such as the ones promoted by the International Committee of Medical Journal Editors (ICMJE). The ICMJE advocates that primary research papers are divided into sections with the headings Introduction, Methods, Results, and Discussion, and sometimes Conclusion. This so-called 'IMRAD' structure, in fact, directly reflects the process of scientific discovery. See section entitled 'Writing your practical report and fuller research papers' in Chapter 3.

Other portions of published papers include the title, abstract, keywords, acknowledgements, references, and individual tables, figures, and legends. Of course, other types of articles, such as case reports, reviews, and editorials, usually follow other formats. Later in your studies you might be asked to write a manuscript for publication (e.g. if you produce original and novel data in your research project). You might be interested to know that different types of studies need to be written up according to very specific and defined formats, in addition to the IMRAD structure. In Table 4.1 we have listed, for your reference, additional reporting requirements for a number of specific research designs.

Table 4.1 Reporting guidelines for specific study designs found on the website of the equator network (Enhancing the QUAlity and Transparency Of health Research; http://www.equator-network.org/)

Reporting guideline	Type of study
CONSORT	Randomized controlled trials
STARD	Studies of diagnostic accuracy
PRISMA	Systematic reviews and meta-analyses
STROBE	Observational studies in epidemiology
COREQ	Qualitative research
ENTREQ	Synthesis of qualitative research
SQUIRE	Quality improvement in health care
CHEERS	Health economic evaluation
CARE	Clinical case reporting

The title, abstract, and keywords of manuscripts are particularly important for helping other people to find a particular scientific paper. This is because these are the main sections of an article that are included in electronic databases (see 'Academic databases' subsection) that we search when trying to identify papers that might be of interest to us. (Things like titles, abstracts, and keywords are what are known as 'metadata'—data that are attached to a given article, which helps search engines to determine whether a given article will be relevant to you, given the search terms you have used.) When you write an abstract it should accurately reflect the article and provide the context or background for the study, including its purposes, procedures, main findings, and conclusions. The abstract should also emphasize new and important aspects of the study–usually within 200–400 words.

If you are using a database to search for original papers (see section entitled 'Academic databases'), the title and the abstract might, in fact, be the only sections of the paper you will at first read. In pharmacy, authors ideally nominate keywords relating to their paper from the medical subject headings (MeSH) list of Index Medicus (see subsection entitled 'Keywords and MeSH headings'); if a suitable MeSH term is not yet available, then authors use other terminology to capture the main topics.

Judging the quality of primary scientific papers

When you find a primary reference that appears, at first glance, to be of interest to you, one criterion you can use to judge its quality is whether the journal uses a peer-review process. Some journals do not adopt a peer-review process, increasing the risk of the publication of studies that are not scientifically robust. But even the process of peer review fails sometimes to pick up things such as a methodological flaw or bias that impacted on data collection and analysis. So how do you judge the quality of a journal publication such that you can be sure of whether or not the information you have found is credible?

One key approach is to use citation indexes and impact factors to help you assess the quality of a publication (which we discuss in more detail in 'Citation indexes and impact factors'). A number of high-impact-factor journals are listed in Box 4.4. The high impact factor of these journals generally tells us that they are respected publications, providing a certain level of

 Box 4.4   Some examples of high-impact-factor journals relevant to pharmacy

- *British Medical Journal*
- *The Lancet*
- *The New England Journal of Medicine*
- *Nature*
- *The Journal of the American Medical Association*
- *Chemical Reviews*
- *Science*
- *Cell*

guarantee that studies published within have been judged to be top-quality research. This is because high-impact journals receive more submissions and can therefore be more selective about the material they accept.

Open-access journals

In the preceding section, we summarized the traditional way in which research is published (see Figure 4.1). The costs of such publications are normally covered through the money generated by individuals or organizations subscribing to the journal (i.e. paying a subscription fee). An alternative model is open-access publishing. Here, the authors make the research available online, via a repository or in a freely accessible journal, and pay for the privilege. This process can bypass a publisher completely, and so can mean that open-access papers are not subjected to strict scientific controls, because their acceptance and publication is based on payment (as opposed to being published as a result of their scientific worth). That said, many leading publishers have open-access journals alongside more traditional subscription-based ones; both types of journal may follow the same, 'traditional' peer-review process. As such, being open-access is not necessarily a sign of poor quality.

There is also a hybrid model, whereby a specific journal may make a subset of its papers available to all in an open-access style if the authors pay for the costs, with others being available to subscribers only. This is because the authors are not paying to have their work published per se but merely paying to make the work freely available on publication.

To double-check whether there are any quality issues with an article you have found you might want to peruse the Directory of Open Access Journals, which is an online directory that indexes and provides access to quality open-access, peer-reviewed journals (http://doaj.org/).

To give access to published work, most UK universities also now maintain an open archive of the peer-reviewed literature produced by their academics. Some may also use this archive to store internally produced technical reports that have not been published elsewhere (or that may be undergoing the review process or are 'in press'—i.e. are awaiting typesetting and final publication). This might therefore be another way for you to obtain papers that you might not be able to access otherwise.

Secondary information sources

Recalling that secondary information sources cover a range of material, we are going to make a distinction here between databases and other publications such as textbooks. Databases are essentially catalogues that you can use in order to locate primary literature (i.e. scientific papers). Textbooks, however, involve authors and editors interpreting and bringing together data from the primary literature by reviewing and rewriting it. Therefore, the two are quite different in terms of their construction, usage, and value.

Databases include commercial academic databases, resource gateways (collections of sites that have been reviewed), and search facilities of Internet search engines such as Google Scholar. In general, databases are searchable resources that index and/or abstract from the primary literature. Most also have alerting systems, which can keep you up to date on any

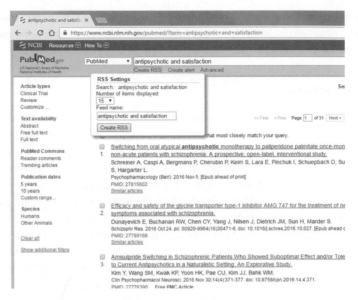

Figure 4.2 A screenshot to demonstrate subscription to an RSS. This screenshot shows the results of a search on PubMed using the keywords 'antipsychotic and satisfaction'. Clicking on the RSS button produces a pull-down menu that allows the RSS feed to be created.

new papers or research published in your area of interest. These are known as a web feed, a data format used for providing you with frequently updated content.

You might yourself be familiar with the web feed known as RSS ('really simple syndication'), which contains either a summary content from an associated website or the full text. As a user you would subscribe to a feed by clicking a link or icon in a browser that then initiates the subscription process (see Figure 4.2). This allows for your subscribed feeds to be checked regularly for new content, meaning downloads are sent to you on any updates found.

Apart from this automatic process, databases are generally searchable and you have to know how to use them to find the information you need.

Academic databases

An academic database is a well-designed catalogue created and maintained by trained personnel for the purpose of keeping and giving access to primary reference sources. Table 4.2 provides some examples of databases relevant to pharmacy.

There are two main types of academic database. A 'bibliographic' database contains information about journal articles, books, and other materials in a summary form called the abstract. A 'full-text' database, however, provides access to the full text of documents electronically. Bibliographic databases can cover a larger breadth of material compared with full-text databases and so might be particularly useful if you are finding it hard to locate the title and abstract of a publication from the existing literature.

The process of creating and adding records to an academic database is known as indexing. Each record in a database describes an item in an organized collection. Box 4.5 outlines

Table 4.2 Examples of databases relevant to pharmacy

Database	Brief description
BioMed Central (BMC) http://www.biomedcentral.com	Database of BMC open-access publications
The Cochrane Library http://www.cochranelibrary.com	A collection of databases, including the Cochrane Database of Systematic Reviews (CDSR)
Embase® https://www.embase.com	A major biomedical and pharmacological database, produced by Elsevier Science
International Pharmaceutical Abstracts (IPA) http://health.ebsco.com/products/international-pharmaceutical-abstracts	Collection of pharmacy literature on drug use and development, pharmacy practice, and education
MEDLINE (see PubMed)	The leading database for biomedical literature, created by the US National Library of Medicine (NLM®)
NICE (National Institute for Health and Care Excellence) Evidence search portal https://www.evidence.nhs.uk	Evidence search provides access to selected and authoritative evidence in health, social care, and public health
PubMed http://www.ncbi.nlm.nih.gov/pubmed	Freely accessible online version of MEDLINE, which contains a number of additional services to MEDLINE
Natural Medicines Comprehensive Database www.naturaldatabase.com	Database of evidence-based, clinical information on natural medicines
PsycINFO® www.apa.org/psycinfo	A database for the field of psychology which covers psychological aspects of related disciplines
REAXYS® https://www.reaxys.com	Chemical database, containing data on structures, reactions, facts, and citations
Science Direct www.sciencedirect.com	Database of Elsevier publications with over 25% of the world's science, technology, and medicine literature
ScienceResearch.com www.scienceresearch.com	A free, publicly available deep web search engine that claims to return high-quality results
SciFinder® www.cas.org/products/scifinder	Information and references, including substances and reactions in chemistry and related sciences
TICTAC www.tictac.org.uk	Visual drug identification other database covering medicines, illicit drugs, veterinary products, vitamins, and others
Web of Science™ https://webofknowledge.com	Database giving access to a range of other databases that can be searched singly or simultaneously

some of the fields contained in a typical record for a scientific paper. Records are maintained 'virtually' in a computer database.

With an academic database you should be able to search systematically the records by using specific search terms to ultimately 'reveal' relevant records from among those held in the catalogue. For example, you might be interested in finding articles on 'drug holidays' taken by patients with attention deficit hyperactivity disorder. An article's keywords should match the terms you would use in your search to help you find it.

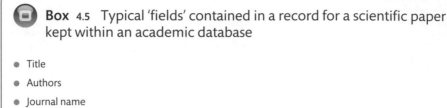

Box 4.5   Typical 'fields' contained in a record for a scientific paper kept within an academic database

- Title
- Authors
- Journal name
- Date of publication
- Page numbers
- Subject classification
- Keywords
- Abstract

When you retrieve a record, the abstract, typically based on the original one from the published paper, should provide the most important information about the item to help you to decide whether you need to look at the full text of the paper. Depending on your university's subscriptions, you might find that the databases you use give direct links to full-text papers that you need to access (see Figure 4.3).

Keywords and MeSH headings

Most journals will ask authors to provide a set of keywords, usually corresponding to MeSH headings, for the purpose of indexing and classification. MeSH is the National Library of

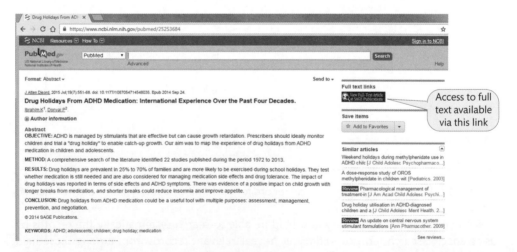

Figure 4.3   A screenshot to demonstrate the facility of clicking on the full-text link to a paper on the page showing the abstract, on a database such as PubMed.

Medicine's controlled phrasebook of vocabulary. Figure 4.4 shows a screenshot of the MeSH interface. MeSH consists of sets of descriptors that are arranged in a hierarchical (and alphabetical) structure, allowing database searches to be carried out at various levels of precision.

At a general level, the hierarchical structures are represented by very broad headings such as 'Nervous System' or 'Psychiatry and Psychology Category'. Further down the hierarchy, more specific headings such as 'Amygdala' and 'Schizophrenia, Catatonic' are found. This means that if you searched for 'Nervous System' in an academic database, your search would return very many papers, but if you were interested in the 'Amygdala' then typing this in would be a better choice as it would limit the number of papers returned (see Figure 4.5).

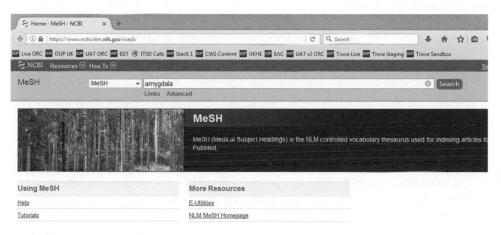

Figure 4.4 A screenshot of the medical subject heading (MeSH) interface.

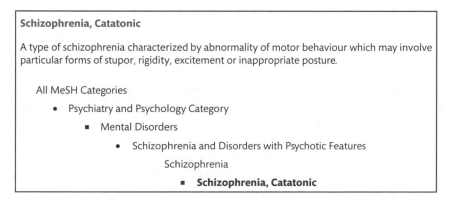

Figure 4.5 A representation of medical subject heading (MeSH) descriptors and headings (adapted from the website of National Centre for Biotechnology Information, U.S. National Library of Medicine).

There were 27,149 MeSH descriptors and over 218,000 entry terms in 2014. Entry terms can help you find the appropriate MeSH heading, even if you do not know it; for example, 'nervousness' is an entry term for the MeSH heading 'Anxiety' and brings you to a page detailing the tree structure for Anxiety. If you learn to use MeSH appropriately, especially when searching PubMed or MEDLINE, then you are more likely to retrieve the papers you need.

Searching academic databases

You might be wondering how you can best search an academic database. Many academic databases now exist, and although their search interfaces might, at first, look very different, similar tools are usually found on each. Some academic search interfaces can look really daunting. For example, the layout might appear overly complex and there might be a very advanced-looking search screen. We will explain here some tips to keep in mind when searching academic databases.

1. Before beginning a new search, you should consider what you already know, what your knowledge gaps are, and the information you require. It is best to have a plan that focuses your search. Select keywords that best reflect the information you need and that narrow the search to a particular subject or topic.

2. When you obtain the results of your search, you should always compare this with the information you originally needed. In fact, unless you are doing a review to find all the information on a particular topic, if you find appropriate material on the first page of your search, then you might stop there.

3. If your search results do not match the information you needed then you should pause and reflect. Think about what you are searching for; can the search be refined by changing keywords, perhaps adding, taking away or replacing them? Your keywords must match the information you need.

The format of the search screen of the database should let you simultaneously search different fields (e.g. author name and journal) by entering multiple keywords in order to retrieve something specific. Sometimes each search entry box on the search screen corresponds to a field. For example, you could enter the search term 'Donyai' in the entry box for author and enter 'The International Journal of Pharmacy Practice' (*IJPP*) in the entry box for journal in order to retrieve this author's full publications in the journal *IJPP* (see Figure 4.6).

Some databases are a bit more complex, showing just one search entry box. Here you would enter 'Donyai P' AND 'International Journal of Pharmacy Practice' to indicate that you would like the search to return articles that combine these search terms. The term 'AND', in this instance, is a *Boolean operator*. If it looks like you might need to use Boolean operators (others include 'OR' and 'NOT') in order to combine your search terms or refine them, then we would strongly advise that you read the help pages available before starting your search.

Not all the fields need be searched during a search exercise, but if you combine search terms and use the fields intelligently then you can better isolate the records you need. For

Figure 4.6 Screenshot showing the PubMed Advanced Search Builder interface, which allows a search to be built by indicating the search field (e.g. author or journal).

example, restricting the keywords to particular fields such as the title or abstract can help focus your search by returning only those articles where the keywords are a prominent feature. You can explore a new database by examining the features that might enhance the efficiency of your search (see Box 4.6).

As stated in the preceding two paragraphs, you might need to use Boolean operators to combine your search terms. The conventional Boolean search operators are 'AND', 'OR', and 'NOT'. They can be used to create a very broad or very narrow search (see Table 4.3).

To make better use of Boolean operators, you can use *brackets* to nest query terms within other query terms. You can also enclose search terms and their operators in brackets to specify the order in which they are to be interpreted. The information within brackets is then read first by the database, followed by the information outside the brackets.

Box 4.6 Checklist for exploring the search interface and other features of an academic database

- How to combine keywords
- How to search in different fields
- How to limit searches
- How to keep track of useful citations
- How to export citations
- What format the information can be viewed in
- How the items might be retrieved
- Whether full text is available
- Whether there is a browse feature for scanning specific journals
- Whether an article's references are also available as links or in full text
- Whether there is a 'cited by' option
- How easy it is to move between articles

Table 4.3 Examples of Boolean operators that can be used when searching academic databases

Boolean operator	Function
AND	Combines search terms so that each search result contains all of the terms. For example, 'pharmacy AND education' finds articles that contain both pharmacy and education
OR	Combines search terms so that each search result contains at least one of the terms. For example, 'medicine OR drug' finds results that contain either medicine or drug
NOT	Excludes terms so that each search result does not contain any of the terms that follow it. For example, 'painkiller NOT paracetamol' finds results that contain painkiller but not paracetamol

For example, when you enter (aspirin OR ibuprofen) AND analgesic, you would expect the search engine to retrieve results containing the word aspirin or the word ibuprofen together with the word analgesic in the fields searched by default.

Sometimes you can also produce brackets within brackets; here, the search engine processes the innermost bracketed expression first, then the next, and so on until the entire query has been interpreted. For example ((paliperidone OR risperidone) AND depot) OR long-acting antipsychotic injections.

Obtaining academic papers

Completing a search will normally result in the retrieval of specific references, but you will probably only want copies of the full academic papers that appear the most relevant to your objective. The quickest and easiest way to determine the relevance of your individual search results is to look through the titles and abstracts. Most databases offer a facility for marking and exporting useful records.

Although we made a distinction earlier between bibliographic databases (those that give access only to titles and abstracts) and full-text databases, most bibliographic databases will, in fact, automatically help you retrieve the full paper through icons such as 'Check for Full Text' and 'View Full Text'. This is because databases can link up with the other subscribed resources available to you when you log in as a member of a university library or similar information service.

However, problems can arise when you try to retrieve a set of references while using a bibliographic database only to find that you cannot get access to the full-text papers because your university does not subscribe to the journals in which the articles are printed.

Full-text resources, however, provide access to full papers. They come from individual publishers, as individual titles, or through subscription agents, who provide a single point of access to electronic journal titles from different publishers and disciplines.

Citation indexes and impact factors

We mentioned earlier that you can use citation indexes and impact factors to help you assess the quality of a publication. Citations are necessary when anyone refer to others' work, as a way of formally acknowledging that the intellectual content you are presenting relates to previously published research (and not your own). A citation should contain sufficient bibliographic information (in the reference list) to allow others to identify uniquely the cited document. An obvious example of bibliographic information for a citation is the reference listed at the end of a scientific paper. For example, the following would constitute a reference: Ibrahim K, Donyai P. Drug holidays from ADHD medication: international experience over the past four decades. *J Atten Disord* 2015;19:551–4.

Commercial databases such as the Science Citation Index® (SCI) and the more comprehensive Journal Citation Report® (JCR) use software to track the total number of times that a journal has been cited by all journals included in the database to return 'total cites' for each journal. In addition, they calculate article counts for each journal covered in the database (each article being a significant item—e.g. a research paper—published in the journal).

Citation and article counts are taken to be important indicators of how frequently current researchers are using individual journals from all available content. From such information, SCI and JCR can then return the impact factor for a journal in any specific year.

Essentially, the impact factor is the average number of times that articles from the journal published in a specific period have been cited by others. Ideally, journals want many citations for each of the articles they produce. The notion, well accepted in the scientific community, is that the higher the impact factor, the 'better' the journal.

Textbooks and other secondary references

Over time, information from primary reference sources becomes assimilated into textbooks and similar publications such as encyclopaedias, drug compendia, and formularies. These publications provide an overview of a topic in a condensed readable form. So, while the authors normally draw on the primary literature for material, textbooks and the like are formatted to suit a particular audience (and, to some extent, the authors' and editors' taste). If you are looking for a particular book then you might find WorldCat® useful (http://www.worldcat.org). This is a cataloguing service that connects to the collections and services of more than 10,000 libraries worldwide.

A wide range of reference sources covering all aspects of pharmacy-related topics exists. They include *Martindale: The Complete Drug Reference*, and the *British National Formulary* (BNF), as well as textbooks covering specific subject areas. Some further examples are provided in Table 4.4.

Textbooks are important for learning established knowledge or accepted information. Writing and producing books is a time-consuming pursuit and many textbooks are updated every 3–4 years to reflect changes in the subject. This inevitably means that it takes quite a long time (circa 5 years) for new research findings to filter into textbooks, so these would not be reference sources to go to for cutting-edge information. In fact, because of the time it takes to write and publish a book, most are no longer completely 'current' even at the point of publication. An important exception is the printed edition of the BNF, which is updated and published as a new edition every 6 months.

Books, compendia, and encyclopaedias, however, are an excellent starting point for learning background information on a subject. Because books are kept on a shelf or in the library, away from the computer keyboard, it is easy to make the mistake of searching the Internet instead of reaching for a good textbook. Remember, books are indexed, and are written to

Table 4.4 Examples of textbooks and compendia relating to pharmacy—see each publisher's website for the latest edition of the publication

Resource	Authors/editors	Publisher
Martindale: The Complete Drug Reference	Alison Brayfield	Pharmaceutical Press
British National Formulary and *British National Formulary for Children*	Joint Formulary Committee; Paediatric Formulary Committee	Jointly by the British Medical Association and the Royal Pharmaceutical Society of Great Britain
Monthly Index of Medical Specialities (MIMS)	N/A	Haymarket Business Subscriptions
The OTC Directory	N/A	Proprietary Association of Great Britain
Chemist & Druggist Directory (C+D)	N/A	CMP Medica
Clinical Pharmacy and Therapeutics	Roger Walker and Cate Whittlesea	Elsevier
Clinical Medicine	Parveen Kumar and Michael Clark	Saunders Ltd
Meyler's Side-Effects of Drugs: The International Encyclopaedia of Adverse Drug Reactions and Interactions	Jeffrey Aronson	Elsevier
Stockley's Herbal Medicines Interactions: A Guide to the Interactions of Herbal Medicines	Elizabeth M. Williamson, Samuel Driver, and Karen Baxter	Pharmaceutical Press
Cytotoxics Handbook	Michael Allwood, Patricia Wright, and Andrew Stanley	Radcliffe Medical Press
Stockley's Drug Interactions	Claire Preston	Pharmaceutical Press
Dale and Applebe's Pharmacy Law and Ethics	J.R. Dale and GE Applebe	Pharmaceutical Press
Basic Clinical Pharmacokinetics	Michael E. Winter	Lippincott Williams & Wilkins
Drugs During Pregnancy and Lactation	Christof Schaefer and Paul W.J. Peters	Elsevier
The Renal Drug Handbook	Caroline Ashley and Aileen Dunleavy	Radcliffe Medical Press

be accessible and easy to understand, so these should be your first port of call for learning new subjects.

Having said that, you must also be aware that the information presented in a textbook is subject to the judgement of the author(s). It is simply not possible for author(s) to search, analyse, or interpret all the relevant information for most books. For example, chapter lengths might dictate less emphasis on certain topics.

Also, books will not be fully referenced. However, none of this should prevent you from using textbooks just because you can search the Internet. Certainly, compared with Wikipedia, good textbooks are an important resource and they should not be ignored.

Table 4.5 Some of the pros and cons of primary and secondary resources

Source	Advantages	Disadvantages
Primary, such as published papers	Contain current, original, and 'cutting-edge' information	Not guaranteed to be without errors or bias You might need to interpret and critically appraise the material yourself It takes time for material in papers to become widely accepted knowledge
Databases	Can unearth primary literature quickly Can give access to high-quality journals Search facilities allow you to pinpoint specific papers Provide facility for routine updates on topics of interest	User needs to have access to primary sources found Can be difficult to navigate and search effectively Searches can return a large volume of relevant material that then needs to be sifted through Cannot browse material (searchable only)
Textbooks and similar publications	Present users with a manageable digest of a vast amount of published information Easy to handle, readable, contain concise information, indexed	Aspects may be out of date almost as soon as published—exceptions include electronic books with frequent updates Information sometimes not comprehensive Do not support full referencing Opinion of author

In addition to books, many students find it helpful to look at YouTube videos to aid their learning. Similar to websites (see section entitled 'The Internet as an information resource') you do have to source reliable information if using YouTube for studying.

Advantages and disadvantages of different reference types

We have outlined the advantages and disadvantages of primary and secondary reference sources in Table 4.5. Read through this table, which is a summary of material already covered.

The Internet as an information resource

If you are part of 'generation Y', born between the 1980s to the early 2000s (or 'generation Z', born later), then it is likely that you will know all too well the ease with which you can access colossal amounts of information on the Internet. But more is not always better: a major pitfall nowadays is relying too heavily on information sources such as Wikipedia. This crowd-sourced database, although easy to discover and understand, is no guarantee of accurate, unbiased, and up-to-date information. Remember that primary sources (and many secondary sources) are reviewed by experts prior to publication, so there is more quality assurance with those. Of course not all of Wikipedia is bad: some of it is very good. It is just that the quality is not consistent throughout because of its crowd-sourced nature.

We are also going to assume that you will be accessing information through the Internet. The Internet in its current form came into being in 1983, so it is over 30 years old at the time of writing this book. Many thousands of documents and other items are added to the web every hour and so it is not possible to create a comprehensive directory of the web. Instead, we would urge you to create your own directory of useful websites.

You can bookmark useful pages using your Internet browser with functions such as 'Favourites' or 'Bookmarks'. You can even organize your bookmarks into folders and subfolders. Social bookmarking websites (e.g. http://delicious.com/) also provide a means of storing personal bookmarks online instead of within the browser, thus enabling you to access and share your bookmark information online.

Searching the Internet

If you have developed a directory of useful websites, you might want to use this to find the information you are looking for. However, merely browsing the Internet (rather than actively searching it) is generally not a very productive way of finding information. With the web, containing trillions of pages, you are unlikely to know where to look for specific information without searching for it. It is essential for you to understand Internet search options, beyond a simple search on Google.

Commercial search engines

Anyone can publish material on the Internet, which, generally, is not controlled or owned by any individual or organization. But there is no central catalogue of webpages that exist online (unlike the table of contents of a book) and no one selects material to create large-scale records. Instead, computers create indexes of the web.

A number of websites, such as Google, provide facilities for searching the Internet. Some are actually set up as web portals to provide a complete resource for everything on the web the authors consider to be worthwhile. Portals display their own editorial material, news headlines, and other up-to-date information, as well as links to commercial partners and paid advertisements. Examples of web portals include Yahoo!, Excite, netvibes, and Bing.

Search engines attempt to search all the text on all the pages of the web. When you type a query, the search engine searches its database for pages that contain words matching your query, displaying the results as a list of links. Search engines rank results according to their own criteria (Google, Yahoo!, Bing, and Ask.com use their own algorithm for returning hits and these can relate to, e.g., the number of quality websites linked to a particular webpage) and so different search engines can give different results for the same query. Search engines are useful for finding obscure information or for some specific activities. Bear in mind, however, that search engines can return a huge number of links that are not necessarily relevant. So it is important to set a time limit when searching the Internet. It also helps to search the Internet effectively. But how can you do this?

Effective use of Internet search engines

Just as it is helpful to have a strategy in mind when performing academic search activities, the same applies when searching the Internet. Think of the most appropriate keywords and subtract any redundant words from your search query. These include words such as 'a', 'an', 'the', 'and', and so on. It can also help if you arrange your search so that the more important search terms are placed first, to give more influence when the results are ranked.

Most search engines provide guidance on their specific 'operators'. For example, Google provides a list of its most popular tools for refining searches on its Googleguide (http://www.googleguide.com). Boolean terms for academic databases were described earlier in the section entitled 'Searching academic databases'. In Google the Boolean terms AND *and* NOT are not used in the traditional sense. For example, Google will automatically link a series of words using the AND operator. If you want to exclude a particular word from your Google search, however, you should leave a space after the word you need and then place a minus sign (-) immediately before the word that is to be excluded. This is useful for words with multiple meanings, like Jaguar the car brand and jaguar the animal. For example 'jaguar speed -car'. In pharmacy you might be interested in searching for training related to Boots (the pharmacy company) but not boots (the type of footwear), in which case you might type 'training boots -shoe' (see Figure 4.7).

You can, however, use the Boolean operator OR in Google by typing OR between two words. Google can also be forced to only include pages with the same words in the same order as what is inside the quotes when you put the word or phrase in double quotes. For example, "Community-acquired pneumonia" will return specific pages that state these words in that order.

Generally, then, you should examine search-engine tools to make the most of any advanced features. Do remember, however, that some public webpages are protected from search engines through use of a file (robots.txt) that blocks access. This normally relates to personal, sensitive, interactive, timely, or premium (subscription, or paid for) content. There are other places, too, that engines cannot sometimes reach; these include commercial data

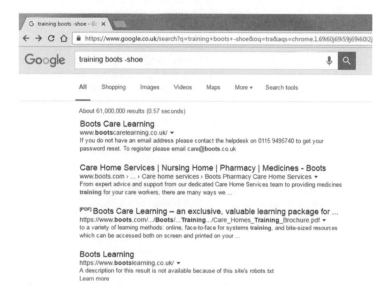

Figure 4.7 Screenshot showing a Google search result with the term 'training boots -shoe' typed in.

collections, or valuable, copyrighted content, information in professional directories, patents, and news articles.

Assessing the quality of information on the web

Anyone from anywhere can publish on the web. There is certainly no editorial process or peer review of every bit of material placed on the web. Therefore, there is every danger that a website can contain unfinished, erroneous, inappropriate, outdated, or even deceptive information. So you should be very careful when using material from the Internet for your studies or later professional practice to inform your work: you have to develop a way of evaluating the quality of the information you find.

When it comes to evaluating the quality of a particular website, we cannot recommend a single quality indicator; it is really up to you to piece together a variety of clues to assess the value of a website on its own merits. The tips listed in Table 4.6 can help you evaluate the quality of information on the Internet and should be used in combination.

Table 4.6 Some tips for evaluating the quality of a website for use in your studies or otherwise

Activity	Purpose
Follow internal links	To find out as much as possible about the resource. For example: what is the scope of the material; who is the intended audience and what is the intended coverage; what is the origin of the information; who owns the website and who is responsible for the content; what is the provenance of the website; what is the involvement of others in the production of material; are there any access restrictions; what is the frequency of updates?
Analyse the URL	To find out where the information comes from and to judge if they are qualified to provide the information. For example, is the web address that of a government agency? That would make it more credible. Who is providing the information and are they qualified to provide the information? For example, who/what is the individual or group that has taken responsibility for the website, are there relevant contact details?
Examine the information contained	To find out the subjects and types of materials covered. Are there any outstanding omissions; what is the audience and what is the level of detail; are there any particular indicators of accuracy (e.g. potential for bias, ability to e-mail corrections); are there any editorial or refereeing procedures; is there evidence of a research basis to the information created; what is the 'main creation date'; what is the frequency and/or regularity of any updating?
Consider the presentation	To find out if the resource is appropriate and whether advertising impacts on the information provided. For example, too many adverts indicate that content might not be impartial. Any access restrictions (e.g. by geographical region, hardware/software requirements)? To find out if the resource is frequently unavailable or noticeably slow to access; is there a registration procedure and is this straightforward; is the available content free or subscription based; what are the copyright statements and copyright restrictions; what is the appropriateness of images and/or advertising; is the site particularly difficult or easy to use; are there user support facilities and/or help information?
Obtain additional information	To find out if the authors are qualified to provide the information. Is the resource well known (e.g. recommended via links), reviewed, and/or heavily used?
Compare to other similar websites	To find out if a resource is unique in terms of content or format.

You can also think about the following criteria when assessing the quality of information on the Internet: presentation; relevance; objectivity; method; provenance; timeliness. The questions to ask here are, do you like the way information is being communicated on a website? Is the information relevant to your needs? Is the information balanced and not being manipulated for, say, financial gain? Is the information opinion-based or scientific? Who has written the work—what are their qualifications? Is the information actually up to date?

User-generated content

User-generated content is widespread on the Internet. Anyone can create content—in stark contrast to peer-reviewed scientific works that are made available by a select group of publishers and editors following editorial standards. Many kinds of user-generated content exist. A particular example is a wiki, which allows visitors to the site to easily add, remove, edit, and change available content, sometimes without the need even for registering. A main example is Wikipedia, a vast online reference work that is written and edited by its users.

Wikipedia has also been the subject of endless debate. Can it be an authoritative reference source if anyone can make changes to it? However, because it can be reviewed by many eyes and be corrected, does it not demonstrate that democratic publishing actually works? Because it is easily accessible and provides wide coverage, you will no doubt use websites such as Wikipedia in preference to good, authoritative textbooks. Our advice is to steer clear as you cannot guarantee the quality of the information on Wikipedia. Instead, try accessing *Encyclopaedia Britannica*, which is actually reviewed and edited and contains a vast body of credible knowledge.

The next chapter, on writing good essays, provides much more detailed information on how to write in your own words, how to cite the literature that you use in your work, and how to reference these using different citation styles.

 Key points

- Information retrieval is about knowing *what* type of information is needed, *where* it might be located, and *how* it might be retrieved.

- Primary information, generated, for example, through scientific enquiry, adds new knowledge to what is already known, and refers therefore to original studies that are normally published in academic journals.

- Authors of original papers normally create accurate, clear reports of their studies for publication and accessing this type of information allows the reader to assess the quality of the work first hand.

- Peer review is considered to be an important part of the scientific process whereby other experts in the field carry out an unbiased, independent, critical assessment of papers describing original studies before they are published.

- Original research papers are traditionally divided into sections headed Introduction, Methods, Results, and Discussion (IMRAD), and Conclusion with some specific research designs following additional reporting requirements.

- The impact factor of a journal is the average number of times that articles from the journal published in a specific period have been cited by others, with a higher impact factor indicating a higher proportion of citations.
- The impact factor of a journal can be used to judge the quality of research papers published within, with a higher impact factor potentially implying higher-quality publications.
- The Directory of Open Access Journals lists peer-reviewed, open-access journals as a marker of their quality rather than mere payment for publication.
- Secondary information draws on primary information and repackages it for different purposes.
- Databases are searchable catalogues that can be used to locate primary literature with bibliographic databases containing information in summary form and full-text databases providing access to full-text documents electronically.
- Textbooks, encyclopaedias, drug compendia, and formularies involve authors and editors interpreting and bringing together data from the primary literature by reviewing and rewriting it—they are a good starting point for learning new material.
- Wikipedia is a crowd-sourced database and although appears to provide some useful material is not peer reviewed systematically and can provide misleading information so it is, overall, better to steer clear of it.
- There is no comprehensive directory of available content on the Internet, but you can create your own directory of useful websites for example using a bookmarking website.
- Presentation, relevance, objectivity, method, provenance, and timeliness can be used as criteria with which to assess the quality of information on the Internet.

 Further reading and references

UK Medicines Information: http://www.ukmi.nhs.uk

Information Retrieval Resources (a comprehensive website with multiple links): http://nlp.stanford.edu/IR-book/information-retrieval.html

5

Writing good essays

Overview

Your university course will almost certainly require you to write essays, potentially as part of an assignment or as part of a formal exam. Some people consider writing good essays to be an art. As well as conveying information accurately you also have to be able to structure and compose your essay in an attractive, even elegant, way. Beyond this, you have to make sure that you have answered the right question and written the material in your own words. Coursework essays can fall prey to copying and *plagiarism*. Knowing how to make use of reference material while maintaining independence in your writing is a key skill to learn and refine at university.

This chapter is all about essays. It will start by considering the nature of essay questions before moving on to explain what generally goes in the introduction, main body and conclusion of an essay. The focus then moves to making effective essay plans and writing a draft. Finally, the chapter explains how to write original material, and cite references appropriately, to avoid plagiarism.

Learning outcomes

You should be able to demonstrate knowledge and understanding of the following after working through this chapter:

- how to interpret an essay question appropriately;
- how to structure and compose your essay;
- how to write in your own words and reference material appropriately.

How to interpret the essay title

The title of an essay specifies the topic(s) it will cover and the problem to be addressed. The 'content words' indicate the topic focus of the essay. For example, you might be asked to 'describe the role of the pharmacist in conducting medicines use reviews'. Here, it seems clear that the topic of the essay is medicines use reviews and that your task is to describe the role the pharmacist plays. The content words are *the role of the pharmacist* and *medicine use reviews*. Essay titles can be more complex though. Consider the following example:

Compare the *educational role* of the *pharmacist* with that of a *general practitioner* in relation to *medicines advice*. Which areas seem *significant* to you and why?

This example has many content words, which have been italicized. The essay title is asking you to examine two professional groups to make a comparison in terms of educational role

Box 5.1   Example essay titles with the content words italicized and the process words emboldened

Explain your opinion on whether *patients in the UK* will be better served by a *system overseen* solely by the *pharmacy regulator* rather than the *criminal justice system*.

List the *symptoms* or *conditions* that may present in a *community pharmacy* that need to be *considered with care* in patients with *diabetes*.

Describe the *epidemiology of bladder cancer*.

in relation to medicines. In addition, the word 'significant' should indicate that only a limited number of areas should be selected for the comparison—rather than the essay being based on boundless points. Box 5.1 contains some example essay titles, with the content words identified using italics.

As well as the content to be addressed, an essay title also indicates the perspective from which you are expected to approach the topic indicated by the content words, which will determine how you organize your writing. This aspect of the essay question is conveyed through the use of 'process words'. For example, an essay question that asks you to 'describe' the role of the pharmacist in conducting medicines use reviews is quite different from one that asks you to 'critique' the role of the pharmacist in conducting medicines use reviews. Process words are typically imperatives, such as assess, explain, describe, compare, critique, delineate, and so on. Consider the example essay titles provided in Box 5.1—the process words have been emboldened.

Returning to the first example:

> **Compare** the *educational role* of the *pharmacist* with that of a *general practitioner* in relation to *medicines advice*. **Which** areas seem *significant* to you and **why**?

Again, the process words have been emboldened. Note that both *compare* and *why* are process words, with 'why' asking you to provide reasons for the particular areas you select to compare the roles. Table 5.1 shows a number of process words and their meaning.

How to organize your essay

Essays can follow different styles but will normally include an introduction, the main body of the essay, and a conclusion. It is very important to read carefully any specific instructions you have been provided to ensure your essay is in the correct form. It is normal practice to write the full essay title at the top of your essay—this is a very good way of reminding you of the content words and the process words to keep you in focus.

The *introduction* is normally no more than one or two paragraphs in length for, say, a 2000-word essay, and defines the main terms and the key topics you will cover and how you will aim to address the essay question.

The *main body* of the essay is the substantive element of your work. Although the rest of this chapter is dedicated to helping you write the main body of the essay, it is worth highlighting

Table 5.1 A number of process words and their definitions

Process word	Meaning
Analyse	Resolve into its component parts, examine critically or minutely,
Assess	Determine the value of, weigh up—see also *Evaluate*
Compare	Look for and show the similarities and differences between examples, perhaps reach a conclusion about which is preferable and justify this
Contrast	Set in opposition in order to bring out the differences—you may also note that there are similarities
Compare and contrast	Find some points of common ground between two or more items and show where or how they are different
Criticize	Make a judgement backed by a reasoned discussion of the evidence involved, describe the merit of theories or opinions or the truth of assertions
Define	Give the exact meaning of a word or phrase, perhaps examine different possible or often used definitions
Describe	Give a detailed account of
Discuss	Explain, then give two sides of the issue and any implications
Distinguish/differentiate between	Look for differences between
Evaluate	Make an appraisal of the worth/validity/effectiveness of something (but not so that it is your *personal* opinion) and give evidence from course materials—see also *Assess*
Examine the argument that	Look in detail at this line of argument
Explain	Give details about how and why something is so
Give an account of/account for	Explain or give the reasons for/clarify
How far/to what extent	Look at evidence/arguments for and against and weigh them up in terms of their value
Illustrate	Make clear and explicit, and give carefully chosen examples
Justify	Give reasons for a point of view, decisions, or conclusions, and mention any main objections or arguments against
Outline	Give the main features or general principles of a subject, omitting minor details and emphasizing structure and arrangement
State	Present in a brief, clear way
Summarize	Give a clear, short description, explanation or account, presenting the chief factors and omitting minor details and examples—see also *Outline*

Adapted from Cottrell S. The Study Skills Handbook. 4th ed. Basingstoke: Palgrave Macmillan; 2013.

here what the main body of the essay is in essence. It is a series of paragraphs that detail the arguments you make and includes the evidence and references that support your statements, and any necessary explanations.

The *conclusion* of the essay is normally a short section that summarizes the main points, focusing on the question but avoiding repetition of material in the introduction. Most essays written as coursework include a reference section, which lists the sources cited within the essay.

Introduction

As explained in the previous paragraphs, the introduction outlines the approach you will take within your essay and provides the reader with an opportunity to see what your essay will include. It is helpful sometimes to use the introduction section to set out your aims, as well as to indicate how your case will develop, by listing your objectives. It is also helpful to give the definitions of any key terms, and also to give a brief description of major debates, or other background information as relevant. The introduction can be up to 10% (as a rough guide) of your total essay word count, depending on the subject and your preference for arranging your material, but it should not normally exceed 10%.

Although an introduction can be an excellent way of helping you to formulate how you might address the essay question, writing it at the start of the process can limit some people. So you might prefer to write the introduction as a final stage instead. Alternatively, you might find it helpful to write your introduction early, then go back and modify it at a later stage, once you have drafted the main body of the essay.

The main part of the essay

In the main part of the essay, you will, of course, be writing the major content of your essay. One key piece of advice is that you should devote each paragraph to one point alone. Taken together, paragraphs make up the topic and argument you are looking to cover. You might recall being taught about 'point—evidence—explanation' in the past. Nonetheless, this is explained here with specific examples. You should use each paragraph not only to state the *point*, but also to provide *evidence* (e.g. citing existing literature) and then an *explanation* of it. The first sentence of your paragraph should also act as a 'signpost' to the reader, so they can understand how the point you are making relates back to the essay question.

Let us use an example to illustrate this point. Imagine answering the essay question '**List** the *symptoms* or *conditions* that may present in a *community pharmacy* that need to be *considered with care* in patients with *diabetes*'.

You may want to focus one of the paragraphs on the importance of diabetic neuropathy in community pharmacy. The point you are trying to make, therefore, is that diabetic neuropathy is one of the conditions that may present in a community pharmacy and that needs to be considered with care. You might make your *point* by writing:

> *One important condition that is likely to present in community pharmacy is peripheral neuropathy caused by diabetes.*

You might then provide *evidence* by elaborating:

> *Over time, high sugar levels in the blood that are associated with diabetes can damage the body's nerves, resulting in diabetic neuropathy. Peripheral neuropathy can present as numbness and tingling in the extremities, a burning or stabbing pain, and*

loss of balance, as well as muscle weakness. Diabetic neuropathy affects 60–70% of people with diabetes, ranging from mild to severe forms of nervous system damage. In addition, 15% will develop foot ulcers and 5–15% per cent of those with diabetic foot ulcers will need an amputation.

Finally, you might *explain*:

This means that diabetic neuropathy is not only a serious condition, but also one that is highly prevalent and therefore likely to present itself within a community pharmacy setting. It is therefore vital for pharmacists to be able to recognize the signs and symptoms of this condition in order to refer patients for further investigation upon suspecting that diabetic peripheral neuropathy is present.

As well as using evidence, you need to support your argument by appropriately referencing the sources that you have used—referencing is covered in more detail in the section entitled 'Organizing and citing references'.

When writing an essay, you should also use the final sentence of each paragraph to link it to the next one. For example, if the next point you were trying to make was about the importance of recognizing diabetic retinopathy, you might *signpost* to the next paragraph by ending the above example paragraph with:

As well as diabetic neuropathy, patients with diabetes can suffer from diabetic retinopathy.

Box 5.2 lists some useful linking words with suitable examples. You should use linking words to weave your essay together and guide the flow of your ideas.

In addition to structuring your essay according to paragraphs in order to cover the 'content' of the essay title, it is important to consider how to address the 'process words'. This is because 'describing' a concept is quite different to, for example, 'analysing' the concept. With reference to Table 5.1, it becomes clear that your essay paragraphs will also have to be written in a way that corresponds with what you are being asked to do with the relevant concepts. For example, if you are being asked to '**Examine the argument that** community pharmacists are not sufficiently competent to recognize the symptoms or conditions that need to be considered with care in patients with diabetes', this is quite different to merely *listing* the relevant symptoms and conditions, as considered above.

In order to *examine the argument*, you would need to consider competing positions. Looking at the essay title, to keep things straightforward, one argument would be that community pharmacists are not competent at recognizing the symptoms or conditions needing special care in diabetes, and the opposing position would be that they *are* competent. Clearly, as a student of pharmacy you might feel impassioned to contest strongly the suggestion in the title. However, far from being asked to take sides, you are expected to make a balanced, dispassionate, and well-argued case for the strength of one position (e.g. that pharmacists are, indeed, competent in the described task) over the other (that they are not). You will need to think about the evidence that you would use in order to make your argument, and how you might compose your argument in the main body of your essay, including what to include

Box 5.2   Linking words with examples

- If you want to **produce a list of ideas** use words and phrases such as: firstly, secondly, finally, or 'the first point to note', 'the second point to note', and so on. For example:

    Firstly, *the early diagnosis and treatment for type 2 diabetes is crucial because it may reduce the risk of developing complications.*

- If you want to **add a point** use words and phrases such as also, in addition, moreover, furthermore, similarly, not only...but also. For example:

    *If blood sugar level is not carefully controlled immediately before and during early pregnancy, there is **also** an increased risk of the baby developing a serious birth defect.*

- If you want to **contrast two points** use words and phrases such as however, although, on the other hand, yet, nevertheless, in contrast. For example:

    *Diabetic patients should aim to do at least 150 minutes of moderate-intensity aerobic activity, every week. **However**, it is important that patients speak with their diabetes care team before starting a new activity. This is because exercise can affect blood glucose levels with the diabetic treatment needing to be adjusted in response.*

- If you want to **illustrate** or **give an example** use words and phrases such as for example, clearly, that is, namely. For example:

    *There are two main types of diabetes, **namely** type 1 diabetes and type 2 diabetes.*

- If you want to **note consequences** use words and phrases such as so, therefore, as a result, consequently, despite, since. For example:

    *In diabetes, some or all of the glucose stays in the patient's blood and is not used as fuel for energy. The body will attempt to remove the excess glucose via the urine. **Consequently**, symptoms of diabetes include urinating more often, especially at night, and feeling very thirsty.*

- If you want to **summarize** or **conclude** use words and phrases such as finally, in conclusion, to conclude, to summarize. For example:

    In conclusion, diabetes is a chronic condition that requires a multidisciplinary approach to its continuing management.

in each paragraph as you progress through your case. This is covered in the section entitled 'Making an effective plan and writing a draft'.

Depending on the 'process words' in your essay title, you might need to take a different approach to what has been described above. For example, if you are asked to *discuss* a topic, you would, again, take an unbiased tone, but you might centre your discussion round comparing and contrasting the different arguments. If you are asked to *explain* something in an essay, you would explore all the elements involved in the concept, again in a dispassionate and even-handed way. Being balanced means that you should use evidence fairly, and not just pick and choose the material that supports your particular line of argument. Ignoring competing material will not make a more compelling case: it will simply portray bias.

In addition to balance, your essay should make clear which elements are factual and which are a matter of opinion. For example, in the essay on community pharmacists' competence, you might find strong evidence of undergraduate and postgraduate training of pharmacists

Box 5.3 Additional tips for writing clear, readable essays

- Use one paragraph per point—do not write long bullet lists or a page or more of text lacking paragraphs.
- Avoid an informal or conversational tone, including contractions such as 'isn't' or 'didn't'.
- Avoid using the first person: instead of 'I think that' say 'It is thought that'.
- Remove redundant words: instead of 'completely necessary' simply say 'necessary'; instead of 'the absolute majority of people' simply say 'the majority of people'.
- Keep your sentences short and succinct—convey only one idea per sentence.
- Use a thesaurus if you need to vary your words, but make sure that the alternative word carries the meaning intended; avoid using 'flowery' words if you are not 100% sure what they mean.
- Use inverted commas around words that are being used in an unusual way.
- Use appropriate vocabulary for the topic or subject.

that suggests relevant capability. However, this would not *prove* for a fact that pharmacists are competent at recognizing and handling the special conditions associated with diabetes— it would simply *suggest* it or support its likelihood. Therefore, you should use phrases such as 'this suggests that...' or 'it is possible that...', and so on, when discussing things that are possibly (but not definitely) true. The University of Manchester hosts a very useful resource that lists academic phrases for explaining causality, as well as other functions; visit http://www.phrasebank.manchester.ac.uk.

Some other key points you should bear in mind when writing essays are presented in Box 5.3.

Remembering that the introduction to your essay should have described clearly what your essay is attempting to cover, defining the essential terminology, from there, in summary, the main body would present your balanced argument, drawing on relevant evidence and with appropriate explanations.

Conclusion

The conclusion of your essay is your opportunity to sum up how your essay has answered the question posed in the title. The conclusion need not be too long—perhaps 5% or less of the total word count. There should be some wording that re-emphasizes the introductory statement you made and also, of course, refers to the words in the title. However, your conclusion should not repeat any examples or word-for-word material from the main body of your essay, nor should it introduce completely new material. Instead, you need to make absolutely sure that your conclusion draws only on the material that you presented in the main body of your essay.

Do take the opportunity to summarize the key components of your argument in a concise and clear way. Make sure that your conclusion is sound in light of the evidence, arguments, and material you have presented. It also helps to be cautious in the conclusion section. Rather than saying 'this proves unequivocally that...', it is much more conventional to say 'therefore the evidence suggests that...', or 'a valid interpretation is that...'. Finally, you could mention the issues that could be considered in the future in light of the evidence found (or not found).

Making an effective plan and writing a draft

The previous section focused on the structure and content of a good essay. However, few of us can be given an essay title and simply start to write, even if we know what the overall structure should be. Instead, an important strategy is to write a plan for your essay. In order to do that you would first need to develop your understanding of the evidence available. Only then can you reasonably decide what you want to include in your essay.

Your first job, then, is to read the essay title and reflect on the type of material you might need to read to inform the content of your essay, and how you might access and collect it, before actually going ahead and doing so. Keep your essay title in mind, to make sure that you are not straying too far from the title. If you have been given a marking scheme for the essay, go through this step by step and plan what you will include in each section, to ensure you have covered every area for which marks will be awarded. You should also check the instructions you have been given for a breakdown of marks for any subsections of the essay. If so, ensure you devote a suitable proportion of your essay to each subsection. For example, if 20% of the total marks will be awarded for the first section of the essay, do not spend 50% or more of your word allocation on writing that section, as you will inevitably run out of words and lose marks elsewhere.

As part of the information retrieval process, you may need to examine and read relevant textbooks, websites, published papers, and lecture notes. Make sure that you keep a complete record of the sources you intend to use to allow you to return to the material and later complete the reference section of your essay.

Making an essay plan

As you gather a sufficient body of material to help you draft your essay, think about which elements you might use to support the arguments you will make—for example, you might paraphrase someone's work, quote a direct sentence, adapt a table, and so on. You can then begin to narrow down this evidence and start to think about how you might actually use the material to answer the essay question. For example, which material might you use as part of the introduction, which for the main element, and so on? It is a good idea then to return to the essay question to make sure that you have not missed any crucial material that will help you make that reasoned and balanced argument. Next, write down your ideas more concretely by making a plan for what each paragraph of your essay will cover.

A plan is simply a rough outline of the structure of your essay. By making a plan, you move from having a mass of ideas to shaping the progress of your argument. It is crucial to again return to the essay title, to make sure that your essay will have the right content and will also address the required process words.

Some people find it helpful to create a mind map of their ideas, others form lists to capture their ideas, and others still write their ideas on sticky notes so that they can re-order them conveniently. Whichever method you use, ultimately the idea with a plan is to commit to a line of argument by outlining the flow of your material.

Writing a first essay draft

Once you have organized your ideas in a plan, the next step is to write the first draft. This can seem a rather daunting prospect. However, your aim with a first draft should not be to produce the perfect essay, but to turn your plan (essay outline) into a series of paragraphs that you can edit at the next stage. Therefore, to start your first draft, simply start to write one sentence at the start of each paragraph to convey the point of that paragraph. Remember that each paragraph should only focus on one point.

Once you have written the first sentence—and remembering the 'point–evidence–explanation' convention—bring together the evidence that supports the points you have made. You will need to decide whether you are paraphrasing material or using quotes from your gathered evidence. Next, write an explanation to make obvious how the evidence supports your claim. Finally, signpost the reader to the next paragraph by using an appropriate linking sentence to complete your current paragraph.

Some students use the total essay word count to assign a set number of words per section (e.g. for introduction, main body, conclusion) then narrow down even further by deciding how many words to devote to each different paragraph or each different idea. Key considerations at this stage are whether the question is being answered through the series of arguments laid out, whether the arguments are dispassionate, supported by evidence and precise, whether the general flow of material is logical, and whether a convincing case is being made.

Creating a second essay draft

Once you have a first draft, the purpose of a second draft is to improve the writing and check that you have not forgotten any major points. You should not normally be looking to conduct a major reorganization of your essay at this stage, although you may find that some restructuring would improve the flow of ideas now that you have everything set out in front of you. If so, now would be the time to make those changes. You should read the material with a view to evaluating whether the essay question is being fully answered in terms of the topics, as well as the process words. You should also check that the sequence of paragraphs is logical and flows well. Of course, if you do make major changes to your essay at this stage, then you may well create more than two essay drafts.

To help with your evaluation, you can ask yourself certain questions about the essay. For example, have you expressed the main ideas clearly? Have you included sufficient examples to support your ideas? Is there a clear structure to your work? Does the material link well together? Have you avoided repetition; check this particularly carefully if you have moved around large chunks of material within the essay.

After that, you should check that the sentence structures are suitable and that your grammar and punctuation are correct. For most essays, it is important to use the right vocabulary, terminology, and notations. Although this proofreading stage might appear to focus on superficial areas such as spelling, use of grammar, and choice of expression and vocabulary, it is nonetheless a crucial final check: the language of your essay is the main means through which you communicate your work, and silly mistakes will create the wrong impression. Thus, we always recommend that students read out their essay either to themselves or (better still) to a friend. This is a final great way of making sure there are no obvious ambiguities or errors, and that the essay is easy to understand.

Writing original material in your own words

So far, this chapter has covered interpretation of the essay title, organizing the essay, and planning and writing drafts. One further important topic is the originality of your writing. When you write an essay it is important to make sure that the reader can distinguish your thoughts and ideas from those of others. Although you are encouraged to refer to other people's ideas, you have to avoid presenting these as your own, which would be considered plagiarism. Plagiarism is acting deceptively to present someone else's material as your own work without acknowledging the original source. If you borrow too heavily from another source and fail to reference the material, you can make it look as though the work is yours as opposed to someone else's.

The best way to avoid plagiarism is to write in your own words, to show that you have read the original material, evaluated and understood it, and can explain it to the reader. Of course, you will still need to credit the original sources that you draw upon using appropriate referencing. We have already stated that a well-written essay uses supporting evidence from elsewhere, perhaps quotations, paraphrasing, or reference to published work. But how do you use quotations, paraphrasing, and reference material correctly? Firstly, we will consider some general principles.

To write in your own words, you should try to avoid mimicking the exact vocabulary employed in the material you are using as evidence for your own essay. Of course, there may be some essential words/phrases you do wish to use, but whenever possible you should not copy the same words into your essay. You are, in effect, expected to reformulate someone else's argument and express it using your own words—for example, by changing the structure of the sentence from the one which you read.

Additionally, you are likely to need only a segment of the original source, as your essay will need its own argument, and other people's work is likely to contain elements that are not needed for your own case. Remember that with 'point–evidence–explanation', you are looking not only to show evidence for your argument, but also to provide your own explanation. This last part will require you to show the relevance of the evidence and indicate how you have formed your conclusion or opinion. This element of explanation must always be written, from scratch, by you.

Using quotations

Sometimes you will find someone else's point so well expressed that you choose to quote their words directly, rather than representing the sentence using your own words. Quoting involves repeating exactly what someone else has said or written. You should introduce the quotation with a phrase of your own and then a comma or a colon. You should then place the sentence or text that you are quoting in quotations marks. For example:

> *It worth noting that the singer will.i.am (2014, p.12) has even commented on the problem of diabetes saying that: 'There are five issues that make a fist of a hand that can knock America out cold. They're lack of jobs, obesity, diabetes, homelessness, and lack of good education'.*

A second rule is to make sure that you have quoted the text exactly as you found it, including any spelling errors and punctuation. If you do find a spelling error or other mistake or anomaly in the quotation, then you can indicate this by using the word [*sic*], placed in square brackets, after the error—*sic* simply means 'thus' from the latin *sic erat scriptum*, 'thus was it written'. Regardless, your quotation should have an accompanying citation so that the reader can see from where the text originates.

Sometimes it is necessary to add some text in the middle of a quotation to add clarity. In such instances you should put square brackets around the added text, similar to what was advocated with the use of the word *sic*. However, you might leave out some words or phrases that are not so relevant from a longer quote and again you should show this by putting ellipses (three dots (...)) where the missing words would have been. For example:

> *'Prescribers should ideally monitor children and trial a "drug holiday" [in those taking medication for attention deficit hyperactivity disorder for longer than a year] to enable catch-up growth. Drug holidays (...) are more likely to be exercised during school holidays'.*

If you find yourself writing a manuscript for submission to a journal (e.g. for publication), you will note that different journals follow a slightly different convention on quotations. It might even be that your university or tutors specify a different set of rules for using quotations. The important thing is to follow a recommended rule consistently.

Paraphrasing

More often, you will find yourself paraphrasing someone else's work rather than directly quoting their work. Paraphrasing is simply rewriting someone else's argument in your own words. The intention here is not to pretend that the work is yours, but to show that you have understood the other person's argument and can present it to fit within your own essay, using your own style of writing. To do this, therefore, you should change the vocabulary of the material where possible, reorganize the structure of the case that was made, and certainly cite the original author whose work you are paraphrasing. For example:

> *The singer will.i.am (2014) believes that diabetes is one of five major threats to North America, among such issues as homelessness and lack of jobs.*

Or you might say:

> *Diabetes is even acknowledged as a problem by a popular culture singer (will.i.am, 2014).*

Of course, although we have cited material from the singer will.i.am, you would normally be expected to cite credible published material unless you were making a very specific point about the public understanding of the threat of diabetes, for example.

Referencing

We have already alluded to referencing in the preceding sections and will cover it in much more detail in the section entitled 'Organizing and citing references'. Referencing is simply a way to acknowledge the source of any quotes, facts, research findings, examples, and other material that you use in your essay. When you use a quotation or mention someone else's work you should include an in-text citation (e.g. giving the author name and publication date) and add the full publication detail in a reference list at the end of your essay. For example, using the Harvard referencing style, you might write:

> *Yet the European guidelines on managing the adverse effects of medication for attention deficit hyperactivity disorder are not in favour of applying drug holidays (Graham et al., 2011).*

Here, the text written in the brackets is the citation: (Graham et al., 2011). The full publication detail would be added to the reference list, here in alphabetical order, for example:

References

Graham J, Banaschewski T, Buitelaar J, Coghill D, Danckaerts M, Dittmann RW, et al. European guidelines on managing adverse effects of medication for ADHD. *Eur Child Adolesc Psychiatry* 2011;20:17–37. DOI:10.1007/s00787-010-0140-6.

Citing an article, for example, in your work ensures that others know when specific material is drawn from the work of others, rather than being your original work.

With electronic material available so easily through the Internet, it can be very tempting to just copy and paste material into your own work. Using references not only ensures that you give credit to whoever created the specific knowledge you refer to in your writing, but it also helps you avoid plagiarism. By contrast, taking other people's work and not showing its source infringes copyright laws and is considered fraudulent. Of course, nobody wants you to reference common knowledge or other information that is universally known, but when you incorporate the work of others into your own, you must acknowledge this. Anything else is considered cheating.

All universities consider plagiarism to be a very serious matter and will investigate potential cases that come to light. Most will use detection software to scan electronically submitted material for evidence of similarity to other works and potential plagiarism.

Although most of this section has explored how to write avoid plagiarism, it is worth concluding with some other important points. When you gather your essay material, make sure that you take notes from original sources. Certainly you should not leave book pages and articles open and in front of you when you write your essay because this can weaken your ability to concentrate on your own writing. You might have to go back to the original sources once you have written your essay to make sure that your writing is not too similar to this material—if it is, then you should certainly amend your essay to distinguish the writing from the source. You should check that you have not inadvertently copied and pasted from other material, including websites. In addition, you should make sure that any assertions you make based on other work or any paraphrasing that you have done includes a citation in the text and a full reference in the reference list.

Organizing and citing references

When you write your essay, you will no doubt want to use a number of different sources in your writing to highlight relevant evidence, as explained in the preceding sections. Although taking notes from a journal article and writing down its source on paper is a useful exercise, most people nowadays use electronic records to store large numbers of retrieved publications and other records for future reference. It is a good idea to use a system for keeping track of the information you amass for later reference. A number of bibliography management systems exist for this purpose; these include RefWorks, EndNote, Reference Manager, and ProCite. These products help you, in effect, to create a personal database of source material. They enable you to import, organize, manage, and export citations, and to create reference lists and bibliographies for your written academic work electronically.

It is also possible to use the in-built feature of Microsoft Word, <References>, to cite and create references for your essay (see Figure 5.1 for a screenshot of this feature).

Some people also use social bookmarking sites such as CiteULike. A social bookmarking site is a service that allows people to add, annotate, edit, and share bookmarks of web documents with others. With experience, you will undoubtedly develop your own way of managing references. Your own university might also recommend and support the use of one bibliography management system so check with library staff if you are unsure.

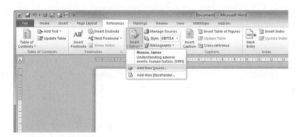

Figure 5.1 Screenshot showing location of Microsoft Word's referencing tool.

Whichever method you use, it is important that you have a systematic way of managing your references. Being organized with your references will help you keep track of what you have gathered and from where. It will save you time locating crucial references (and the original source if need be). In addition, inputting the right information into a management system will make sure you can provide a full and accurate reference list, and, crucially, allow you to change the style of the citations and referencing, if needed, with relative ease.

When writing an essay, you should make sure that you have checked which referencing style is required by your university or tutor. A number of referencing styles exist for citing retrieved information, and most academic institutions and publications have standardized requirements. Whichever style of referencing you use, you would be expected to have recorded some standard details relating to the sources you have used. These include the author(s), title of the work, the year it was published, where it was published, and so on. Some of the more widely used styles are listed in Box 5.4.

Whatever style you use, accuracy, clarity, and consistency are the key factors when citing information sources. Two of the common referencing styles, the Harvard and the Vancouver styles, are worth examining in detail here. With the Harvard referencing style you are expected to cite the surname of the first author, as well as the year of publication, separated by a comma and placed in brackets, within the appropriate sentence in your essay. If you already mention the surname of the author within your sentence, then you need only place

---

 Box 5.4 Common referencing styles

- American Psychological Association (APA), sixth edition:

  Thompson Coon, J., Abbott, R., Rogers, M., Whear, R., Pearson, S., Lang, I., . . .Stein, K. (2014). Interventions to reduce inappropriate prescribing of antipsychotic medications in people with dementia resident in care homes: a systematic review. *The Journal of Post-Acute and Long-Term Care Medicines*, 15, 706–718

- Chicago Manual of Style, 15th edition:

  Jo Thompson Coon, et al. "Interventions to Reduce Inappropriate Prescribing of Antipsychotic Medications in People With Dementia Resident in Care Homes: A Systematic Review," *The Journal of Post-Acute and Long-Term Care Medicines* 15 (2014): 706–18.

- Harvard:

  Thompson Coon, J. et al. (2014). Interventions to Reduce Inappropriate Prescribing of Antipsychotic Medications in People With Dementia Resident in Care Homes: A Systematic Review. *The Journal of Post-Acute and Long-Term Care Medicines*, 15, pp. 706–718.

- Modern Language Association (MLA), seventh edition:

  Thompson Coon, Jo, et al. "Interventions to Reduce Inappropriate Prescribing of Antipsychotic Medications in People With Dementia Resident in Care Homes: A Systematic Review." *The Journal of Post-Acute and Long-Term Care Medicines*, 15, (2014): 706–18.

- Vancouver/ICMJE:

  Thompson Coon J, Abbott R, Rogers M, Whear R, Pearson S, Lang I, et al. Interventions to reduce inappropriate prescribing of antipsychotic medications in people with dementia resident in care homes: a systematic review. J Am Med Dir Assoc. 2014; 15: 706–718.

the date within the brackets, straight after the author's name. If you use a quotation, the Harvard referencing style dictates that you also cite the page number of the reference, where the quotation was found. For example:

> *Diabetic neuropathy affects 60–70% of people with diabetes, ranging from mild to severe forms of nervous system damage (Tindall, 2010).*

> *According to Tindall (2010), diabetic neuropathy affects 60–70% of people with diabetes, ranging from mild to severe forms of nervous system damage.*

> *It is worth bearing in mind that 'diabetic neuropathy affects 60–70% of people with diabetes, ranging from mild to severe forms of nervous system damage' (Tindall, 2010, p. 3).*

There are some other general rules for making in-text citations using the Harvard style, which are worth mentioning here. One rule relates to citing publications with more than three authors, which is shown in Example A by the use of 'et al.' (meaning 'and others') after the surname of the publication's first author, Tindall.

Example A:

Diabetic neuropathy affects 60–70% of people with diabetes, ranging from mild to severe forms of nervous system damage (Tindall et al., 2010).

Another rule is where you have cited multiple publications by the same author published in the same year, as illustrated by Example B. Here, you would place an 'a' immediately after the publication year for the first citation and 'b' for the next, and so on.

Example B:

Diabetic neuropathy affects 60–70% of people with diabetes, ranging from mild to severe forms of nervous system damage (Tindall, 2010a). In addition 15% will develop foot ulcers and 5–15% per cent of those with diabetic foot ulcers will need an amputation (Tindall, 2010b).

Finally, where you have cited multiple sources for the same statement (Example C), you would simply write all the sources within the same bracket following the statement.

Example C:

Diabetic neuropathy affects 60–70% of people with diabetes, ranging from mild to severe forms of nervous system damage (Tindall, 2010; Hughes, 2014; Patel, 2016).

You then need to list all the sources you have used within a reference list at the end of your essay. The Harvard referencing style sees the references arranged in alphabetical order. The general Harvard reference style is shown in Figure 5.2.

There are different referencing conventions for different publication types, with published journal articles being referenced differently to books, using the Harvard style. A book would be referenced: Author, A. (year of publication) *Title of Book*, place of publication, publisher.

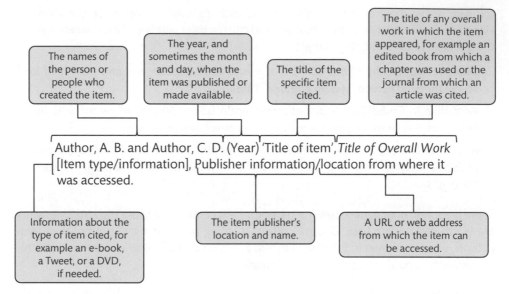

Figure 5.2 The general Harvard reference style explained.

For example:

Donyai, P. (2012) *Social and Cognitive Pharmacy: Theory and Case Studies*. London: Pharmaceutical Press.

A journal article would be referenced: Author, A. (year of publication) 'Title of article', *Title of Journal*, volume number (issue/part number), page number(s) (abbreviated to p. or pp.).

For example:

Ibrahim, K., & Donyai, P. (2014). Drug Holidays From ADHD Medication: International Experience Over the Past Four Decades. *Journal of Attention Disorders*, 19, pp. 551–68.

This book will not provide examples of every reference type (e.g. book, journal article, thesis, website, etc.). This is for two reasons. Firstly, bibliography management systems (e.g. RefWorks, EndNote, Reference Manager, and ProCite) and even the <References> feature of Microsoft Word are all equipped to produce the reference list for your essay automatically and according to the relevant referencing style. Secondly, there are now online citation tools available that show you how a reference should look according to the desired style (e.g. website vs book reference). These online sites include EasyBib and Citation Machine. Box 5.5 summarizes example reference formats for the Harvard style.

Most biomedical journals follow the Vancouver/International Committee of Medical Journal Editors (ICMJE) referencing style rather than the Harvard style. With the Vancouver/ICMJE referencing style a number is placed within the sentence at the point where you cite someone else's work, with subsequent citations following in numerical order. This number can be inserted in brackets or as superscript text, and, if appearing at the end of a sentence, either before the full-stop or immediately after it. The exact format depends on the guidelines you are provided with for your essay, or the guidance you are asked to access (e.g. for journal manuscript submission). You should then list all the sources you have used within the

Box 5.5   Some general formats for references, including punctuation for the Harvard style

Standard journal articles

List the authors then the publication year followed by article title:

Author, A. B., et al. (Year of publication). Title of article. *Journal name*, <volume(issue)>, pp. <page number(s)>.

Example:

Donyai, P., et al. (2011). British Pharmacy Professionals' Beliefs and Participation in Continuing Professional Development: A Review of the Literature. *International Journal of Pharmacy Practice*, 19, pp. 290–317.

Books

Where the book is written by personal authors (rather than editors):

Author, A.B., et al. (Year). *Book Title*. Edition [abbreviated to ed.—only include this if not the first edition] Place of publication: Publisher.

Example:

Donyai, P. (2012). *Social and Cognitive Pharmacy: Theory and Case Studies*. London: Pharmaceutical Press.

Homepage/websites

Name of source or authorship (Year). *Title of web document or webpage* [type of medium—e.g. online] (date of update, if available) Available at: <website URL> [date accessed]

The Pharmaceutical Journal (2015). *Careers* [online] Available from: http://www.pharmaceutical-journal.com/careers/ [Accessed 4 May 2016].

reference list at the end of your essay in order of citation (i.e. in number order and therefore in the order they appear in the text).

For example you might write:

In clinical practice, inadvertent 'human failures' have been categorized as **thinking errors (action as planned: rule-based and knowledge-based mistakes) and** *action* **errors (action-not-as-planned: action-based slips and memory-based lapses) [4].**

Then the fourth reference in your list would be:

4. Reason J. Understanding adverse events: human factors. Qual Health Care. 1995;4:80–89.

The Vancouver style dictates a different way of writing the reference list compared with the Harvard (and indeed other) referencing styles. This includes the way in which the author names are listed, the punctuation use, the use of italics, and so on. Box 5.6 includes some example reference formats for the Vancouver style.

This brings to an end the chapter on essays. The key points listed here are a reminder of some of the important elements covered. The next chapter provides information on a different type of assessment, namely verbal in-course assessments, including poster and oral presentations, as well as oral examinations.

Box 5.6   Some general formats for references, including punctuation for the Vancouver style

Standard journal articles

List the first six authors followed by et al. Most journals carry continuous pagination throughout a volume, so the month and issue number may be omitted:

Author AB, Author BC, Author DE, Author FG, Author HI, Author JK, et al. Title of article. Journal name [abbreviated journal name]. Year of publication;volume:page number(s).

Example:

Donyai P, Herbert RZ, Denicolo PM, Alexander AM. British pharmacy professionals' beliefs and participation in continuing professional development: a review of the literature. Int J Pharm Pract. 2011;19:290–317.

Books

Where the book is written by personal authors (rather than editors):

Author AB, Author CD, Author EF. Book title. Edition [abbreviated to ed.] Place of publication: Published; Year of publication.

Example:

Donyai P. Social and cognitive pharmacy: theory and case studies. 1st ed. London: Pharmaceutical Press; 2012.

Homepage/Websites

Name of website [Internet]. Place of publication: Organization; Year [date accessed]. Available from: website URL

PJOnline [Internet]. London: The Pharmaceutical Journal; 2015 [cited 2015 July 19]. Available from: http://www.pjonline.com/

 ## Key points

- You should read the essay title for the 'content words'—what you should cover—and the 'process words'—how to organize your writing.

- It is important for you to understand the meaning of different process words so that you can style your essay to meet the requirements of the essay.

- Make a rough outline of the structure of your essay to guide you with writing the first draft.

- Your introduction should define relevant terms and describe the key topics you will cover and your general approach to answering the essay title.

- You should organize the main body of your essay by devoting one paragraph to one point, providing relevant evidence and an explanation for your point.

- You should end each paragraph by signposting to the next paragraph or to another relevant part of your essay.

- You should support the arguments you make in your essay by citing suitable references.

- Your conclusion should summarize the main points you have covered without repeating the same material.

- Use a first draft to map out your essay outline and the second draft to refine and proofread your work.
- Write your essay in your own words using quotations, paraphrasing, and in-text citations to reference your work.
- Use a bibliography management system to organize and cite your references.
- Use the referencing style recommended for your essay with consistency and accuracy.

 ## Further reading and references

Academic Phrasebank (2016). *The Academic Phrasebank 2016 Enhanced Edition* [downloadable pdf file]. Available from: http://www.phrasebank.manchester.ac.uk [Accessed 4 May 2016].

American Medical Association (2015). *American Medical Association (AMA) Manual of Style* [online]. Available from: http://www.amamanualofstyle.com/ [Accessed 4 May 2016].

American Psychological Association (2015). *American Psychological Association (APA) Publication Manual* [online]. Available from: http://www.apastyle.org/ [Accessed 19 July 2015].

Anglia Ruskin University (2016) *Harvard System* [online]. Available from: http://libweb.anglia. ac.uk/referencing/harvard.htm [Accessed 4 May 2016].

Citation Machine: http://www.citationmachine.net/ [Accessed 19 July 2015].

CiteULike: http://www.citeulike.org/home [Accessed 19 July 2015].

EasyBib: http://www.easybib.com/ [Accessed 19 July 2015].

Harvard College Writing Center (2016). *Strategies for Essay Writing* [online]. Available from: http://writingcenter.fas.harvard.edu/pages/strategies-essay-writing [Accessed 30 April 2016].

Modern Language Association of America (2012). *Modern Language Association (MLA)* style [online]. Available from: https://www.mla.org/style [Accessed 4 May 2016].

The University of Chicago (2010) *The Chicago Manual of Style 16th Edition* [online]. Available from: http://www.chicagomanualofstyle.org/home.html [Accessed 19 July 2015].

University of Reading (2016). Develop your essay writing [online]. Available from: https://www.reading.ac.uk/internal/studyadvice/StudyResources/Essays/sta-developessay.aspx [Accessed 30 April 2016].

US National Library of Medicine (2013). International Committee of Medical Journal Editors (ICMJE) Recommendations for the Conduct, Reporting, Editing and Publication of Scholarly Work in Medical Journals: Sample References [online]. Available from: http://www.nlm.nih.gov/bsd/uniform_requirements.html [Accessed 19 July 2015].

6

Perfecting verbal in-course assessments

 ## Overview

This chapter is about verbal assessments: it is likely that you will be required to undertake several of these during your pharmacy degree. We will look at a range of types of verbal assessment, including poster and oral presentations, 'vivas', and objective structured clinical examinations (OSCEs). Students often find these quite challenging, so we will describe the basic requirements and some useful techniques for both the verbal and written elements of these assessments.

As with many aspects of learning, different universities (and even academics within the same university) approach things differently, so the first thing to remember is to look carefully at what is expected of you. This means looking at the guidance provided for you by your university (e.g. module descriptions or assessment guides), which will give you information about the knowledge and skills that they want you to demonstrate, and how they will judge these. Marking criteria will often be made available for these assessments, so familiarize yourself with these as part of your preparation.

As with all assessments, preparation is key. This is especially relevant for verbal assessments, particularly if you are someone who gets very nervous in such situations. This chapter will dissect these assessments and give you some useful hints and tips along the way.

 ## Learning outcomes

You should be able to demonstrate knowledge and understanding of the following after working through this chapter:

- how to structure, compose, and deliver a presentation;
- how to design a poster;
- how to prepare for a viva;
- what an OSCE is, and important points to remember when undertaking one.

Giving a presentation

Presentations are a commonly used method of assessment within pharmacy degree programmes, owing to the importance of pharmacists being able to synthesize information and communicate it effectively. They allow academics to assess a range of skills, including your ability to identify, collate, and interpret appropriate information (usually from a range of sources), and deliver this information in a concise, organized, and clear manner, taking account of the needs or 'level' of your audience. It is likely that your assessors will be looking at the structure of your presentation, the content that you have included, how you visually present that content, and how you verbally communicate it to the audience. They may also assess how you handle any questions asked during, or after, the presentation.

Although preparing a presentation may seem like a daunting task, thinking about the following aspects should help you to achieve success.

Content and illustrations

In order to deliver an effective presentation, preparation is essential. When planning the content of your presentation, remember to think about the assessors' intentions: what are they looking for? What is the assessment brief? Have you been provided with guidelines regarding how to design or structure your presentation?

Common topics of presentation include:

- giving an overview of a disease state, or a particular treatment;
- describing a patient case study or plan for their pharmaceutical care;
- giving an account of a research project and its findings.

Clearly, the content of these will differ, but the overall rules for a good presentation are similar. It is likely that, as part of the assessment brief, you will be allocated a topic to cover within your presentation. However, you will still need to think about what specific content to include—how much should you cover and to what level of detail? One aspect that is important to consider as part of this is your audience. Specifically, there are four questions about your audience to consider, as illustrated in Figure 6.1.

A successful presentation will be tailored to the needs of the audience: if the content is too simple, they may get bored and 'switch off'; if it is too complex, they may find it difficult to understand and, again, are likely to stop listening. Assessed presentations will usually be delivered to your peers, which should make it relatively easy to decide on the level of content to include. However, you will also need to bear in mind your assessors and what they are

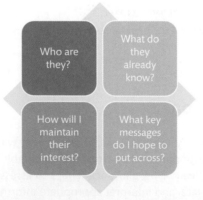

Figure 6.1 Questions to consider about your audience when planning a presentation.

looking for, in order to achieve the good marks that you are probably hoping for! The assessors will usually be the lecturers that have taught you the content, but they may be academics from another section, or perhaps even other students, or a combination of these. Think about what existing knowledge of the topic they are likely to have, and keep this in mind at all times—this will help you to decide how much explanation you need to give and the level of complexity to include. Remember to check whether the assessment brief instructs you to design the presentation for a particular audience—for example, a group of patients, or health care professionals.

Key messages

When considering what content to include in your presentation, think about what key messages you would like your audience to leave with. This will help you to keep your presentation 'on theme' and avoid rambling. Depending on the length of the presentation, you should usually aim for no more than five of these 'key messages', which are clearly highlighted to the audience and, where relevant, reinforced with examples or scenarios where they may be applied. For example, in a presentation about preventing coronary heart disease, you might wish to highlight the importance of providing lifestyle advice. This could be reinforced with images relating to a healthy lifestyle, or a short case study about a patient and the relevant advice that could be given to them.

Presenting your content

It is likely that you will be using presentation software, such as Microsoft PowerPoint or Prezi. The way you design your presentation will depend, to an extent, on the functionality of the software that you are using. We will look at some hints and tips for using this type of software later in the chapter.

Structuring your presentation

When structuring your presentation, think of it like a story—having a beginning (the introduction), a middle (the main content), and an end (the conclusion).

The *introduction* helps to set the scene of your presentation, outlining the topic that you will be covering, signposting the different sections that you will move through, and, hopefully, gaining the audience's attention. It is usual to have a title slide, containing the title of your presentation and the name(s) of the presenter(s).

Some approaches that you could use to try to engage the audience from the start of your presentation include using a patient case study, an interesting or amusing fact about the topic, or a question. Depending on the type and requirements of the presentation, you may then wish to include the aim and/or an outline of what you intend to talk about.

When thinking about the *main content* of your presentation, think about the required duration of the presentation and tailor the quantity of content and level of detail accordingly. It is important to try to ensure that the presentation follows a logical order, as this will help the audience to follow the flow and 'make sense' of what you are talking about. You will find this easier if you split the content that you wish to include into sections. If your research has

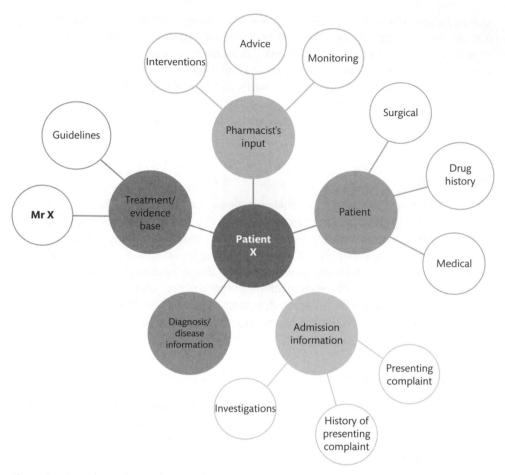

Figure 6.2 Example mind map of content for a presentation about the care of a patient while in hospital.

left you with a lot of content that you are not sure how to divide up, you may find it useful to write out or 'mind-map' the presentation (see Figure 6.2 for an example relating to a presentation about a particular patient and their care while in hospital). Remember to bear in mind the marking criteria or other requirements of the assessment, to ensure that you include any specified content, and reference your sources of information in line with the guidance provided by your university (see Chapter 5 for more information on referencing).

When designing your presentation, ensure that you make each section clear (e.g. with a section heading) and think about how you will move from one section to another. For example, depending on the quantity of content, you may wish to sum up the key message(s), ask for any questions relating to the section, or refer back to your outline slide to introduce the next section.

Illustrations

When writing your content, consider how you can illustrate your points with images or diagrams. Don't go overboard—make sure that they are relevant and appropriate to the message that you are trying to get across. Jokes are usually best avoided! When adding images or figures to your presentation, check that the audience will be able to read them clearly. If there is too much information, consider summarizing the key points and showing these instead, providing more detail verbally. Alternatively, you could provide a document for the audience to refer to. Remember to leave yourself time in the presentation for an explanation of these figures and also for any additional examples that you may wish to include.

The *conclusion* is the end of your story, summarizing and reinforcing the key messages that you are trying to put across, and bringing the presentation to a close. At this point, many presenters will thank the audience for their attention, and encourage them to ask any questions that the presentation may have raised.

Using presentation software

Whichever presentation software you use, it is important to use it correctly—this can be the difference between a successful presentation and the rather-less-desirable 'death by PowerPoint'. The key is for the slides that you produce to complement your presentation and not distract from it; including too much animation, for example, can be distracting for the presenter, as well as the audience. Similarly, overuse of 'fancy' slide transitions can also be detrimental. When designing your slides, think about the following:

Use a large, clear font	Avoid lots of text or long sentences
Use pictures, photographs, simple graphs/tables	Avoid excessive/unnecessary images and animation
Aim to keep away from the edges of the slides	Avoid small or complex images
Use bullet points where possible—ideally no more than 5–6 per slide	Avoid using too many colours

Good and bad examples of the use of PowerPoint are given in Figure 6.3.

It is usually a good idea to include a title slide, containing the presentation title, your name, and, especially if presenting project work externally, the organization's logo.

When deciding on a colour scheme, remember that light colours (e.g. yellow text) on a white background can be difficult to read.

Generally, most people use dark text (e.g. black) on a light background. If possible, check your presentation beforehand using a projector to see if the text and images can be seen clearly from the back of the room.

Presenting and presentation skills

So, you've written your content. Now let's think about the presentation itself. Alongside the preparation that is essential for a successful presentation, practice is also important. It can be

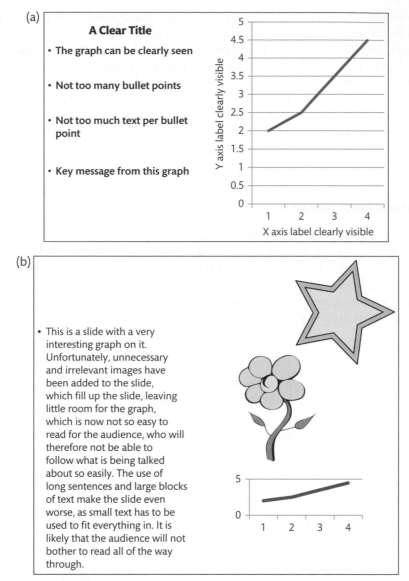

Figure 6.3 Slide design: (a) the good, (b) the bad (and the ugly).

particularly useful to read through the presentation out loud—this is the best way to practise your presentation skills. Rehearsing in this way will help in a number of ways:

- having a good knowledge of the material will boost your confidence and reduce your reliance on reading from your notes, which will improve your presentation style;
- it will help you to identify any sections that do not flow naturally;
- it will give you the opportunity to practise your pronunciation of any words with which you are less familiar (e.g. tongue-twisting drug names);
- it will give you an indication of how long your presentation will last.

You may find it helpful to practise in front of friends or family to get feedback, or using a mirror or video so that you can observe your body language.

Some aspects of communication to think about to ensure a successful presentation are given in Table 6.1.

Should I use notes?

Most presenters will use some form of notes when presenting. If you are very familiar with the content of your talk, you may decide to present without notes: this will show that you are confident and knowledgeable about your topic. However, if you lose your train of thought you may find it difficult to get back 'on track'.

If this is the first time that you have presented, you may be tempted to write yourself a script to learn or read from. While this will help to ensure that you do not forget anything that you want to say, you will probably find it difficult to engage effectively with the audience, as it will be difficult to maintain eye contact without losing your place in the text.

A common compromise between these two options is to use notecards, or printed copies of the presentation slides with annotations. These contain the key points relating to each slide or section and act as prompts for what you want to say. This method gives the benefits of helping you to remember your key messages and keep your presentation well structured, while still allowing you to maintain a good level of eye contact with your audience. This can work particularly well if you practise using them beforehand, as you will probably find that you need to adapt them to fit the way you deliver the content of the presentation.

If you do read from notes, ensure that you do not lift your notes up so that they obscure your mouth or face. This will make it harder for your audience to hear what you are saying, and will act as a 'barrier' between you and your audience.

Group presentations

Presenting as part of a group can be much less daunting than presenting alone. However, delivering an effective presentation as a group requires careful planning, to ensure that each individual has the opportunity to contribute and responsibilities are distributed fairly. The presentation should be split into sections that are of a similar size in terms of timing and information to be covered. Ideally, each person should speak once only, as having too many sections or changes in speaker will make the presentation seem disjointed.

Rehearsing as a group will be important to help ensure that your presentation flows well, avoids unnecessary repetition, and to promote a smooth handover between presenters. As each new speaker takes over, they should clearly state what aspect they will be covering, as this will help to give structure.

You should also think about how the group will position themselves during the presentation; it is important that those who are not speaking do not distract attention from the person presenting. This may be facilitated by having the speaker standing slightly in front of the rest of the group, who should focus their attention on the person presenting and avoid excessive movements and fidgeting.

Table 6.1 Communication hints and tips to help you present effectively

Do	Avoid
Appearance	
Do check the dress-code for the presentation	Avoid looking scruffy! This can affect the audience's perception of you as a presenter
Try to maintain an outwardly confident appearance. The audience will feel more at ease if you appear calm and in control	Try to avoid nervous habits, such as fiddling with your hair, or repeatedly clicking a pen—this can be distracting for the audience
Think about your body language. For example, try to maintain an open stance—this will help you to look (and feel) more confident	Avoid crossing or folding your arms in front of you, as this can make you look nervous, or 'closed off'
Do feel free to move. You do not need to stay still for the whole presentation	Avoid pacing up and down, or swaying from one leg to another. Also try not to use exaggerated gestures, e.g. waving your arms or hands around
Connecting with the audience	
Do try to look around the whole audience, making eye contact with them	Don't forget those at the back of the audience—make them feel included and involved
If you are feeling nervous, focusing your attention on those who appear interested in what you are saying can help to increase your confidence	Don't hold prolonged eye contact with individuals, as this can make them feel uncomfortable
Try to position yourself to the side of the projection screen, so that you do not block anyone's view	Avoid reading from the projection screen, as this will usually require you to turn away from the audience and put your back to them
At the end of the presentation, thank the audience for listening	Don't just present to the assessors or your friends!
Your voice	
Try to project your voice so that those at the back of the room can hear you clearly. You may wish to ask the audience if they can hear you if you are unsure	Avoid shouting, as this will be uncomfortable for the audience, and for you
Speak clearly, at a rate that allows your audience to understand you easily. Be prepared to repeat or explain any points that the audience does not understand	Try not to speak too fast. This is easier said than done, especially if you are nervous. If, during your practice, you identify that you have too much content for the time available, cut down the material—don't just try to talk fast to fit it all in
Varying the pitch and tone of your voice will help to hold the audience's interest	Avoid speaking in a flat, monotonous way
Use pauses to give the audience time to digest an important point or key message. You may also find it useful to include pauses between different sections of the talk, to highlight the end of one section and the beginning of the next	Avoid uncomfortably long pauses, or 'er' and 'um', as these can disrupt the flow of the presentation and show a lack of confidence
Face the audience at all times while speaking—this makes a real difference to how well they will be able to hear you. Keep your hands away from your mouth	Don't talk to the projection screen
Do practise your pronunciation of any words with which you are less familiar, e.g. difficult drug names or medical terms	Avoid exaggerated pronunciation—don't feel that you have to 'put on a voice'—your natural speaking voice will be fine

Tips for dealing with nerves

The first thing to remember when trying to overcome nerves is that you are not alone! Everyone gets nervous before a presentation, even those that are used to doing them. So what can you do to feel less nervous?

- Prepare and practise. As mentioned earlier, the more you do beforehand, the better you will know your material and the more confident you will feel. This is especially important for group presentations—make sure that each member of the group knows which section they will be contributing to, and how it relates to the content being delivered by others.

- If possible, visit the venue beforehand—this will allow you to familiarize yourself with the layout of the room, the materials that are available (e.g. whiteboard, flipchart), and how to use the equipment (e.g. computer and projector). Think about where you will stand; using a pointer device or 'clicker' will give you greater flexibility and allow movement. You may also want to try out the acoustics of the room—how far will you need to project your voice?

- Have a back-up plan in case of problems with the equipment. For example, if you are using a computer and projector, you may wish to take some paper copies of your slides so you can distribute them to your audience (or at least those assessing you) if the projector malfunctions.

- Take a few deep breaths before the start of your presentation. Remember to give yourself pauses to breathe during the presentation—this will help to control your nerves and also improve your ability to project your voice and speak clearly.

- Maintain a natural and upright stance, facing the audience, with your feet slightly apart (e.g. hip-width). Avoid pacing and large gestures or movements.

Dealing with questions

One aspect that presenters often fear the most is the questions they may be asked during, or at the end of, their presentation. During this part of a presentation you may feel that you are no longer 'in control', which can be a worrying feeling. However, the question-and-answer (Q&A) section of a presentation is very important, as it allows the audience the opportunity to clarify any information that they did not understand, and allows the assessors to probe your knowledge and understanding in greater depth.

We said at the beginning of this chapter that preparation is key, and this also holds for the Q&A part of your presentation. The questions that you are asked by the audience will be related to a particular aspect of your presentation, so having a clear theme or topic, and re-searching this thoroughly during your preparation, will greatly increase your ability to answer any questions effectively.

When reading the assessment brief, remember to consider the time that is allocated, es-tablish whether questions are included as part of this, or are in addition, and plan accord-ingly. When designing and writing your presentation, decide whether you would prefer the audience to ask questions as you go, or whether you would prefer them to save any questions until the end; inform them of the approach you have decided upon during the initial outline of your presentation. It is generally a good idea to invite the audience to ask questions when you have reached the part of your presentation at which you had planned to take them.

Answering a question

So, you've been asked a question. What next? Consider the following three steps:

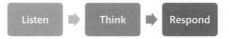

Listen carefully to the whole question. Try to avoid making assumptions about the question that is being, or might be, asked, as you may miss important information, or misinterpret the question. Concentrate on the person asking the question and let them finish before starting to formulate your response.

Once the question has been asked, give yourself some time to *think*—don't feel that you have to jump in with a response. Check that you have interpreted the question correctly and ask for clarification if you need it. You may find it helpful to paraphrase the question, or relay your understanding of it, back to the person who asked it. Consider whether any of the information in your presentation will help you to answer the question—referring back to the relevant section may be useful.

When you *respond* to the question, try to keep your answer concise, and direct it to the audience, as well as the person who asked the question, so that everyone is included in the discussion. Make sure that you answer the question that was posed, and not what you had hoped would be asked. The careful listening mentioned in the first step is important for this. At the end of your response, you may wish to check with the person who asked the question that you have answered appropriately. When being asked questions, it is often easy to feel that you are being criticized—it is important to put such feelings to one side and answer all questions in a calm and professional manner.

If you are asked a question to which you do not know the answer, don't panic! It is usually better to admit that you are unsure, perhaps suggesting that you will find out the answer and respond to them at a later time, rather than to try to 'blag' your way through.

Being asked questions should be seen as a positive thing—if the audience is asking you questions, it usually means that they listened to what you were saying and found your presentation interesting.

Preparing a poster presentation

As an alternative to delivering a presentation with a slideshow, you may be asked to present your work as a poster presentation. Your assessment brief will usually state the basic format requirements for the poster—for example, the overall size, the font that you should use, and sometimes the section headings that you should include. Ensure that you take note of these, as the ability to follow instructions often forms part of the assessment.

Think carefully when designing your poster—the biggest challenge will most likely be how to fit all of the information that you wish to include into the space that you have available, without necessitating the use of a microscope in order to read the text. Figure 6.4 shows an

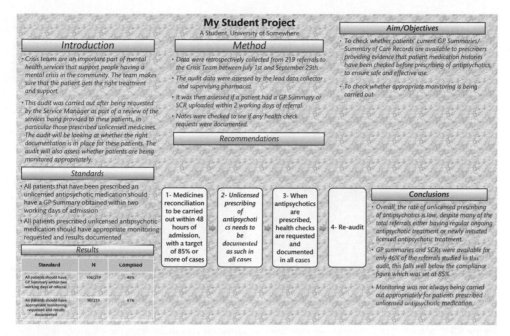

Figure 6.4 Example of a poorly designed poster. The key issues are (1) the poor flow and poor use of space; (2) the poor placement of figures and diagrams, and their lack of titles; (3) the distracting background; and (4) the inconsistent fonts used.

example of a poster with several design flaws. Read on to find out what to remember when producing a poster, and things to avoid.

Content

As mentioned in the previous subsection, check your assessment brief for any specified section headings. Posters will generally include: title and author(s), a brief summary, introduction, the 'main body' of the content (for a research project this would include methods and results), a conclusion, and references.

You will need to be selective about what you include; for example, for a research project, only include the results that relate to the main findings of your work.

Appearance

Visual impact is likely to form a large component of the marking scheme for a poster presentation, so think carefully about the design of your poster, remembering that empty space is as important as the text and images that you include—it helps to give a poster a clear flow. Keeping a good balance between text, images, and the space around them will ensure that the poster is easy to read.

Plan the overall layout of your poster before you start, using a logical flow of information—this should normally be from top to bottom and left to right, unless instructed otherwise.

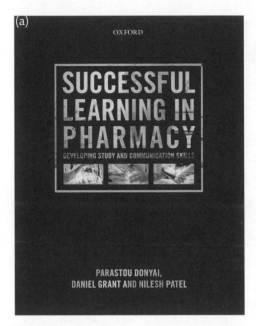
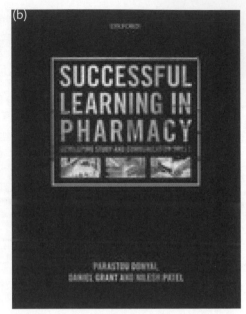

Figure 6.5 Examples of pictures at (a) high resolution and (b) lower resolution. Note the difference in quality of appearance.

Images should be of a high enough resolution to print well at a large size—pictures from the Internet are often not of high enough quality to be used for this purpose. Low-resolution pictures may appear unclear, grainy, or even pixelated (see Figure 6.5). Remember to take account of copyright issues where relevant; you may need to credit the source (e.g. giving the artist's name, image title, and website from which you obtained the image) or obtain permission to use the image. University libraries can often provide advice in relation to copyright if you are unsure. Remember to follow any instructions that you have been given in relation to the inclusion of illustrations, tables, and graphs.

Fonts should be in accordance with your assessment brief. If not specified, choose a clear font (often called 'sans serif'), as they are easier to read. Avoid using multiple fonts throughout, as this can make your poster look messy; use larger font sizes and bold text to identify important words or headings.

Colour should be used carefully—it is usually best to use a simple colour scheme. Avoid difficult-to-read colours, as described earlier in the chapter, such as yellow text on a white background.

Finally, proofread your poster carefully. It is all too easy to miss typographical or spelling errors.

The poster presentation

The way that the poster presentation itself takes place will depend on the assessment brief. You may be working as part of a group and be asked to present information relating to a particular section of the poster; you may be working on your own and be asked to provide a summary of the poster contents; or you may just be required to respond to questions asked by those reading your poster. Whatever format the presentation takes, the tips that we discussed earlier in the chapter for presentations will also apply here, so take a look back at the earlier sections, including how to handle being asked questions.

Performing in tests such as objective structured clinical examinations and vivas

In this next section, we will take you through two types of oral assessments: vivas and OSCEs.

Vivas

A 'viva' (more properly known as a viva voce, from the Latin meaning 'with the living voice') is an oral assessment often carried out in relation to project work or research, and is used to examine your deeper understanding of a topic, or range of topics, and your ability to communicate this understanding. It may also be used in some universities as a method for assessing students that are on the borderline between classifications after final examinations are complete.

The duration of a viva can vary considerably, depending on what is being assessed; they may only last 10–15 minutes for an undergraduate project but up to 3 hours for a PhD. Your assessment brief should give you an indication of the duration. There will normally be two assessors, one of whom may be your supervisor.

Preparing for research project vivas

When preparing for a viva relating to a research project that you have completed, a good starting point for preparation will be to re-read your project report. Think about what the project was trying to achieve, the background evidence to the topic area, your methods, findings, and conclusions. You should also be prepared to justify your conclusions and discuss any weaknesses of your project design; consider yourself the expert and be prepared to demonstrate and defend this point. Some examples of questions that you may be asked are as follows:

- Why is this topic important?
- What were the key findings?
- What challenges did you encounter?
- What are the limitations?
- What would you do differently next time?

If you do not understand a question, do not be afraid to ask your assessors to repeat it for you.

Vivas in relation to final classifications

In some universities, students whose final marks lie on the borderline between two degree classifications (e.g. between a 2:1 and a 2:2), or whose performance may have been affected by specified mitigating circumstances, may be invited to a viva. The important thing to remember with this type of viva is that you will not lose marks as a result of a poor viva—you will keep the marks you have already gained. The two outcomes of a viva are to move up to the next classification, or for your classification to remain the same.

In this type of viva, it is likely that one of the assessors will be a member of staff from another university, who will be carrying out the viva as part of quality-assurance processes. You should have been provided with clear information about what to expect from your viva—if not, ask well in advance of the date of the viva. Topics will vary, but the aim of the viva is to provide the examiners with evidence of the breadth and depth of your knowledge and understanding of subjects from across the degree programme. It is likely that you will also be asked questions regarding any large pieces of work that you have completed—for example, a final-year dissertation or research project.

This type of assessment is difficult to prepare specifically for, other than the advice given above in relation to project-based questions. Think about the modules that you have undertaken, in particular any that you have found more difficult—it may be worth revisiting these.

Tips for viva voce examinations

- Wear appropriate clothing—it is usual to dress smartly for this type of examination.
- Listen carefully to the questions that you are asked. If you are unsure, politely ask the assessor to repeat the question.
- You may find it helpful to have some 'holding phrases', such as 'In my opinion...', to give you some thinking time when answering difficult questions.
- Try to answer each question fully, avoiding 'yes' or 'no' answers.
- Stay calm. Some of the questions that you are asked may seem difficult—this is to be expected as the examiners will be aiming to push you to assess the extent of your knowledge.

OSCEs

OSCEs, or objective structured clinical examinations, are often used in pharmacy degree programmes as a form of assessment that requires the integration of a range of skills, including communication, clinical, and practical skills. They may be used formatively (to give you feedback on how you are progressing), or summatively (a formal, 'credit-bearing' assessment). This type of assessment usually takes the form of a series of short 'stations', in which you will encounter different scenarios designed to mimic situations that may be encountered in the workplace.

Examples of OSCE scenarios include:

- calculations;
- responding to symptoms;
- clinical assessment of a patient;

- providing advice to a patient—relating to a particular medicine or device, or health-promotion/lifestyle advice;
- medicines history taking/medicines reconciliation;
- assessing prescriptions for legal validity and clinical appropriateness;
- dispensing a prescribed item.

As you will see from the examples given, OSCE stations may be 'manned' (in which you undertake role play with a member of the OSCE team, an actor, or an 'expert'/simulated patient), or 'unmanned' (e.g. a dispensing task). However, the assessment will often comprise a combination of these two types of station. Some assessments will include 'rest stations', which are intended to give candidates time to catch their breath. You may also be given a 'reading station', where you are given time to read some material which you will need to use during the next station.

You will move around the stations, each of which will usually be of a similar duration (perhaps 10–15 minutes). As you enter the station, you will be provided with the scenario. An example of a scenario that you might be given for a responding to symptoms consultation is as follows:

'You are the pharmacist working in a community pharmacy. A man in his 40s approaches the pharmacy medicines counter and asks to speak to you.'

Some stations may then include some preparation time for you to gather your thoughts and think about the scenario given, while others may require you to start immediately. OSCEs can be logistically complicated, so it is important that you listen carefully to the instructions that you are given. An example of how a series of OSCE stations might be put together is shown in Figure 6.6.

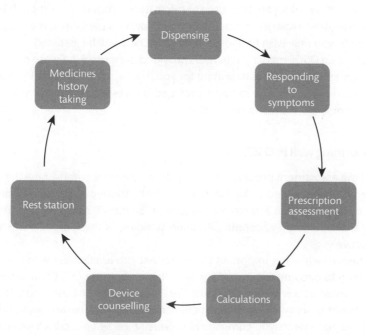

Figure 6.6 An example of a set of OSCE stations

The way in which OSCEs are assessed varies from university to university, so it is important that you familiarize yourself with the guidance that you will have been provided with by the person leading your module. Look carefully at the marking criteria and the knowledge and skills that are being assessed. For manned stations, communication and consultation skills will often form an important part of the assessment—you will not only be assessed on *what* you say, but also *how* you say it: for example, using appropriate language and terminology, building a rapport with the patient, acting professionally and showing empathy, and following a logical approach to the consultation.

The marking scheme may incorporate both the technical and consultation skills aspects of the task in one, or they may be separated into a *technical or analytical checklist* and a section marking your consultation and behavioural skills. A *global assessment* is also sometimes used, to grade how you managed the task as a whole; this may be described as a clear pass (the task being appropriately managed), a borderline pass (the task only just being satisfactorily managed), or a fail (the task being unsatisfactorily or incorrectly managed). The global assessment may be used to take account of errors made that may lead to patient harm—a candidate may achieve a high score on other aspects of the marking scheme but still fail that task overall if something that they said or did could cause harm.

The pass mark for an OSCE assessment may be chosen as a set score (e.g. an average of 40% or 50%), or it may be calculated using 'standard setting', which can be carried out in a variety of ways. In one method, called borderline regression, the assessors identify candidates that they consider to be at the borderline, and calculate the pass mark after the assessment has taken place, through statistical methods using their marks. In another method, the Modified Angoff method, prior to the OSCE the assessment panel make predictions of the proportion of minimally competent students (i.e. those who would just pass) that would achieve a particular criterion. These values are then used to calculate the pass mark. Although the method by which the pass mark is assigned should not affect how you perform in the OSCE, as part of your preparation you may wish to find out how your OSCE will be assessed.

An example of an OSCE marking scheme is provided in Figure 6.7. Please note that a wide variety of schemes is used, so it is important for you to ensure that you are familiar with that used in your own university. The example provided is a 'responding to symptoms' scenario for a male patient in his 40s with a sore throat.

Tips for performing well in OSCEs

Understand the assessment process—including the assessment criteria, how the session will run, whether you are allowed to take in notes or make them during the examination, and so on. Find out if there is an assessment syllabus or 'blueprint' outlining the range of tasks or scenarios that you might encounter. An understanding of these aspects will help you to prepare effectively.

Get experience—while it is important to ensure that you are familiar with the assessment criteria, it is easy to become too focused on this. Remember that OSCEs are designed to assess how you would deal with simulated real-life situations, so the best preparation you can undertake is to obtain as much practical experience as possible; for example, through making good use of the placements you complete at university, and gaining work experience. Such experience will help you to perform well in your OSCEs but will have much wider benefits to you as a future pharmacist.

Technical checklist

The Student:	Achieved
Gathering information	
Asks who is the patient	
Asks how old is the patient	
Asks what are the symptoms	
Asks if the patient also has a cold, cough, or difficulty swallowing	
Asks how long have the symptoms been present	
Asks if the patient has tried anything already	
Asks if the patient smokes	
Asks if the patient is taking any medication	
Asks if the patient has any medical conditions	
Asks about allergies	
Option/management strategies (including patient education)	
Advises patient to stop taking carbimazole and see GP straightaway	
Explains reason for referral is that the sore throat may be an adverse effect of carbimazole	
Advises patient that they can use lozenges until they see the GP	
Advises to suck ONE lozenge every 2 to 3 hours	
Advises not to use more than 12 lozenges in 24 hours	
Gives non pharmacological advice–up to 3 marks	
E.g. avoid food or drink that is too hot as this could irritate your throat, eat soft food, suck hard sweets, ice cubes or ice lollies, avoid smoking and smoky environment, drink plenty of fluids (cool or warm)	
Total Percentage %	

Consultation skills

	0	1	2
Greets patient in appropriate manner	No greeting or disengaged	Gives name or role	Engaging and welcoming, gives first name and role
Explains purpose of the consultation or need to ask questions	No explanation or rushed/muddled	Broad description	Clear and concise description of what is involved. Checks patient understanding
Verbal expression	Poor or confusing. Reads entirely off PIL	Checklist approach to consultation, rather than engaging with patient	Good fluency, grammar, vocabulary, tone, volume and modulation of voice, rate of speech and pronunciation
Non-verbal expression	Fails to engage with patient. Significant time spent reading resources	Some effort to engage patient	Good use of eye contact, gesture, posture, shows interest

Fig 6.7 cont.

Checks patient understanding of information	Not done	Minimal effort, checks at end of consultation	Checks understanding throughout discussion
Summarizes information provided	Not done	Adequate, may be rushed	Clear and concise
Provides opportunities for the patient to ask questions	Not done	Offers opportunity to ask questions	Questions encouraged throughout consultation
Brings the consultation to a conclusion	Does not finish	Concludes, but is rushed/abrupt	Concludes in a professional manner
Total percentage %			

Global assessment

Fail	Borderline	Pass
Management of task would cause serious patient harm or death	Student manages the task with minimal competence	Student appropriately manages the task
0%	Max 40%	

Please give details if Fail or Borderline:

OSCE review panel comment/ decision:

Figure 6.7 An example of an objective structured clinical examination marking scheme, showing the technical checklist, consultation skills marking scheme, and global assessment.

Practice—get as much practice as you can before the examination. You may find it helpful to carry out role-play scenarios with your friends. If you have been provided with sample stations by your module lead, make use of them. Some stations may allow use of specified reference sources; if this is the case, ensure that you are able to use those sources of information efficiently and effectively. Check whether you are expected to bring your own references and any requirements associated with this; ensure that any references you do take with you are well organized and meet the specification (e.g. are you allowed to tab useful pages or highlight text?).

Read the information/scenario carefully—you may be provided with an outline of the scenario prior to entering the station. Read this carefully and use it to help guide your approach to the station.

Stay in role—you will usually be asked to act as though you are a qualified pharmacist. You should aim to stay in this role throughout the OSCE station and not ask questions of the examiner as a 'student'.

Remember the scenario—the person with whom you will be consulting may be a member of staff, an actor, or a patient representative. However, it is important that you bear in mind the scenario; for example, the 'patient' may be an 80-year-old woman, in which case it would not be appropriate to ask if she is pregnant!

Remember the basics—in the stress of the examination, it can be easy to forget the basics that would normally come naturally; for example, introducing yourself, confirming the patient's details, checking for allergies or medical history, and closing the conversation. These will often form part of the assessment criteria for manned stations. If you find consultation skills difficult, you may find it helpful to work through the learning provided by the Consultation Skills for Pharmacy Practice website (see 'Further reading and references' for details).

Listen carefully—at manned stations, listen carefully to what you are being told by the person with whom you are consulting—they may be giving you important information. Try to avoid just going through your questions in a tick-list manner; listen and adapt your consultation accordingly.

Manage your time—you will usually have a limited amount of time in which to perform each OSCE station. Keep an eye on how long you have remaining and adapt your approach to avoid running out of time.

Finally, **don't panic**—try to keep calm, as this will help you to perform to your best. If a particular station doesn't go well, try to put it to the back of your mind and focus on the next station. It is often possible to perform poorly in a station but still do well overall.

 Key points

- Read the assessment brief and ensure that you understand what is expected of you.
- Manage your time effectively.
- Do not be tempted to guess or 'blag' if you are unsure.
- Think about the person or audience you are communicating with, and their needs and interests. Listen carefully to what they are saying or asking.
- With all of the types of assessment described in this chapter, nerves can have a major effect on your performance. Preparing well will help you to feel in control.

 Further reading and references

Centre for Pharmacy Postgraduate Education (2014). *Consultation Skills for Pharmacy Practice* [downloadable pdf document]. Available from: http://www.consultationskillsforpharmacy. com/docs/docb.pdf [Accessed 4 June 2016].

Evans BW, Kravitz L, Lefteri K. Pharmacy OSCEs: A Revision Guide. London: Pharmaceutical Press; 2013.

Presentations:

Your university will most likely have information available on its student webpages about preparing and giving presentations and poster presentations.

See http://www.reading.ac.uk/internal/studyadvice/StudyResources/sta-seminars.aspx for an example (accessed 9 August 2015).

You may also find the Businessballs website useful as an easy-to-understand source of information and advice about giving presentations. See http://www.businessballs.com/presentation.htm (accessed 4 June 2016).

Vivas:

Your university may also have information available about viva examinations. See http://www.stars.rdg.ac.uk/viva.html for an example (accessed 9 August 15).

Applying critical thinking and critical writing

 Overview

You will be expected to perform at different levels as you progress through your pharmacy degree course. While the learning expected of you in the first and second years of your course is likely to be relatively straightforward, the demand, complexity and depth of learning, and your independence will increase in the latter years. For example, when you are assessed in the earlier years, you might be expected to demonstrate evidence of knowledge and comprehension. However, later in your course you are likely to be asked to apply your knowledge and understanding to specific cases, for example by analysing a problem, or evaluating some published evidence. This is because your pharmacy degree is preparing you for a range of cognitive abilities and skills which you will need to employ in order to practise effectively as a pharmacist. On completing your degree, you are expected to be able to critically evaluate, interpret, and synthesize pharmaceutical information and data; recognize and analyse problems and plan strategies for their solution, and so on.

This chapter, then, is all about higher-level critical thinking and critical writing— activities that are much needed for learning in the latter years of pharmacy degrees, including for writing reports and dissertations. Firstly, we will define what is generally understood by critical thinking. Secondly, we will examine ways in which you can start to examine other people's work with a critical mind. We will conclude with how to write using a critical voice.

 Learning outcomes

You should be able to demonstrate knowledge and understanding of the following after working through this chapter:
- how to read material with a critical mind;
- how to write with a critical voice.

What do we mean by 'critical thinking'?

Degree courses become progressively more complex as students progress from the first to the final years. We know this, in part, as a result of the work of Benjamin Bloom, who devised a framework for classifying what educationalists expect of students as a result of teaching them. Bloom's original taxonomy of educational objectives provides definitions for six major categories: knowledge, comprehension, application, analysis, synthesis, and evaluation. Bloom's taxonomy has since been revised, resulting in the re-working of the six major categories as: remembering, understanding, applying, analysing, evaluating, and creating (Box 7.1).

Bloom's taxonomy serves a useful purpose for our discussions. The idea, then, with a degree course such as pharmacy is for you, as the learner, to move beyond simple knowledge

---

 Box 7.1   Structure of Bloom's revised taxonomy

Structure of Bloom's revised taxonomy

1   **Remember** Retrieve knowledge from long-term memory
   - Recognizing/identifying
   - Recalling/retrieving

2   **Understand** Construct meaning from instructional messages, including oral, written, and graphic communication
   - Interpreting/clarifying/paraphrasing/representing/translating
   - Exemplifying/illustrating/instantiating
   - Classifying/categorizing/subsuming
   - Summarizing/abstracting/generalizing
   - Inferring/concluding/extrapolating/interpolating/predicting
   - Comparing/contrasting/mapping/matching
   - Explaining/constructing models

3   **Apply** Apply a procedure to a familiar task
   - Executing/carrying out
   - Implementing/using

4   **Analyse** Break material into its constituent parts and determine how the parts relate to one another and to an overall structure or purpose
   - Differentiating/discriminating/distinguishing/focusing/selecting
   - Organizing/finding coherence/integrating/outlining/parsing/structuring
   - Attributing/deconstructing

5   **Evaluate** Make judgements based on criteria and standards
   - Checking/coordinating/detecting/monitoring/testing
   - Critiquing/judging

6   **Create** Put elements together to form a coherent or functional whole; reorganize elements into a new pattern or structure
   - Generating/hypothesizing
   - Planning/designing
   - Producing/constructing

Adapted from Krathwohl DR. A Revision of Bloom's Taxonomy: An Overview. Theory Pract. 2002;41(4):212–17.

acquisition (level 1 of Bloom's taxonomy) to understanding and applying the knowledge (levels 2 and 3), to analysis and synthesis of material (levels 4 and 5), and then to evaluation of material and creation of new material (level 6), from the first to the final years. Critical thinking relates to the latter stages, especially the evaluation and creation of material.

Thinking critically about other people's work applies to almost anything you read while studying for your degree if the text has involved the author *pursuing a line of reasoning*. This means that critical thinking applies just as well to book chapters, Internet articles, and newspaper clippings as it does to primary scientific publications.

An important point to note is that Bloom's taxonomy is often used in order to define learning objectives, and also the criteria for assessments. Criteria for assessment relate to the 'process words' explained in Chapter 5 on essay writing. While certain process words such as define, describe, identify, label, name, outline, reproduce, recall, and so on, which are used to set out an assessment task might relate to the earlier levels of Bloom's taxonomy, process words such as interpret, defend, distinguish, explain, discuss, formulate, judge, contrast, compare, and so on relate to the more complex, higher levels. Thus it becomes essential not only to understand the meaning of these verbs, but also their relationship to Bloom's taxonomy, if essay and exam questions are to be answered in a way that demonstrates the expected level of learning.

The *Oxford Dictionary of English* defines critical thinking as 'the objective analysis and evaluation of an issue in order to form a judgement'. In Chapter 5 we introduced you to a range of terms (process words) that relate to critical evaluation, including *analyse, assess,* and *evaluate*. In this chapter, we aim to examine these concepts in more detail, beginning with the idea of reading and thinking critically about other people's work.

Examining other people's work with a critical mind

At university, reading should move far beyond the mere ingestion of information (as one might do with a work of fiction, for example). The whole purpose of a university education is to develop you, the student, into an independent learner who can think and scrutinize material for yourself. To do this, you need to first develop effective ways of reading and understanding a range of subjects. It seems an obvious point, but most of what you read at university should be new to you. Before you can start to critique any material, you need to engage with what is being conveyed at an academic level. To help you with this first step, we have listed a range of tips for effective reading in Table 7.1.

What is conveyed in Table 7.1 can be summarized as a *quick* then *slow* approach to engaging with your reading material. The quick element (scanning, skimming) relates to a surface assessment of the text and whether it might be relevant to your needs and therefore worth spending your time on. This is an important skill that you must develop if you are to use your time effectively. The slow element relates to a process of actively engaging with the text in more depth not only to understand it, but also to question its validity. It is this latter process—questioning the validity of information being presented to you—which lies at the heart of reading and thinking critically about other people's work. Of course, only once you have understood your material can you begin to think critically about what you have read.

Table 7.1 Tips for effective reading

Recommendation	Explanation
Formulate the purpose of your activity	When you read a paper, or a book chapter, always do this having clearly thought about the exact purpose of the activity. This will help you prioritize what to read and also guide you in what to look for specifically. For example, are you reading a book chapter to supplement your lecture notes, or because you need essential background information before writing an essay?
Scan the material for relevance	Gain a general overview of the material by quickly looking over the entire work; how many pages, how many sections, what subheadings, images, tables, which particular topics? This will help you assess the potential relevance of the work for your specific purpose. For example, does the book chapter look as though it is covering your subject of interest in sufficient depth or breadth?
Skim the material by reading key elements	Read the first paragraph or introduction to the text, as well as the last paragraph or conclusion; read the first few sentences of other paragraphs of potential interest. This will help you assess the potential relevance of specific elements of the work. For example, which parts of the book chapter look as though they might be specifically suited to your purpose?
Actively engage with the text	Use a range of techniques to not only 'see' the words on the page, but also to understand the meaning of what is being conveyed; for example, highlight or underline words, annotate the text, use sticky notes, make separate notes, or make mind maps. This will help you think more deeply about what you are reading. For example, is it actually clear to you what is being said?
Question the material	This is about the context of what you are reading: who has written the work, when did they write it, who was the audience, why was it written, how does it link with existing/other knowledge? This is a good step towards critically processing what you are reading. For example, is what you are reading actually a reliable source of information?

In a nutshell, then, thinking critically is an analysis of the material in terms of its key components such as how well the argument is made. You might want to think about the main points of the argument, the claims being made, the evidence used and the conclusions reached. Thinking critically is about exploring the similarities and differences with other published work; how the paper or chapter compares with what you have learnt or read before; and whether the ideas conflict with other arguments or support and build on them. So, far from taking what you read for granted, you are expected to interpret what you read and examine its validity and reliability.

One of the key processes involved in critical evaluation is the assessment of material for its relative merit. Through this process you should decide whether the arguments presented are worthwhile and whether they contribute to what is already known. Some of the questions to ask are as follows:

- Who has produced the material? What is their expertise and experience?

- Why has this work been put together? Is there a hidden agenda or has someone been paid to put forward a particular point of view?

- When was the paper written? What was the received wisdom at the time and have ideas evolved over time?

- Where was the work published? Is the source reliable and does it provide confidence about the scientific merit of the work?

A useful way of conducting a critical evaluation is to apply a framework to the way you approach your assessment of the work. We are going to introduce here the idea that you can conduct critical evaluation at a microlevel, that is, examining a sentence or a paragraph; and then at a macrolevel, that is, examining an entire research paper or book chapter. One way of doing critical evaluation at the microlevel is to examine the material in terms of the coherence of the arguments and the evidence being presented. So what do we mean by this?

The *coherence* of an argument is about the line of reasoning used, whether the conclusions drawn are valid, whether any assumptions have been made, and whether alternative claims have been considered. The *evidence* for an argument is about the type of material used to support the claims, whether they are appropriate, recent, or important, whether the evidence conflicts with other evidence, and whether methodological issues might cast doubt on the strength of the evidence. We will examine an extract of text from a research manuscript to illustrate this point—remember that we are completing critical evaluation at a microlevel here:

> *The short-term adverse effects of methylphenidate can be very harsh for patients and their families because this medication can suppress appetite and growth of children and cause sleep problems (Authors et al., 2004).*

In terms of the *coherence* of this argument, the authors are stating that:

(a) Methylphenidate has side effects.

(b) Methylphenidate can suppress appetite and growth in children.

(c) Methylphenidate can cause sleep problems.

(d) These side effects can be very harsh for patients and their families.

On the face of it, the line of reasoning used here seems coherent: the medication causes a range of short-term side effects, and these can be very harsh for patients and their families—the conclusion seems valid. However, on closer examination, there are assumptions being made here. For example, children are normally prescribed methylphenidate for attention deficit hyperactivity disorder, a disorder which itself is associated with sleep problems, before medication is started. The extract does not consider this alternative point.

Turning now to the *evidence* for the argument, the extract uses one reference to support the entire claim. Firstly, the reference is rather dated, from 2004. In addition, the reference is placed right at the end of the sentence—it is unclear, therefore, which element of the argument the reference is supporting, the existence of the side effects, or the experience of parents and their children, or both. An alternative way of writing this text might be:

> *A number of researchers have documented the unpleasant experiences of patients and their families with methylphenidate (Authors et al., 2004; Authors et al., 2012), which is known to be associated with short-term adverse effects, including suppression of appetite and growth, as well as sleep problems (British National Formulary, 2016). It has to be noted, though, that the experience with sleep is difficult to unravel because unmedicated children with attention deficit hyperactivity disorder also suffer from sleep problems (Author, 2009).*

As well as critiquing distinct elements of the material you are reading (a study or paper), you will be looking to critique the whole piece. One way of doing critical evaluation at the macrolevel is to assume different levels or 'modes' for evaluating the text. This is to help you frame whether you are critiquing the *conduct of a study*, the *type of study* being presented, or the study's *arguments*. These can be thought of as *mode 1*: a within-perspective critique; *mode 2*: a between-perspective critique; and *mode 3*: a meta-perspective critique. The idea of these modes comes from reading material one of the authors encountered while studying psychology with the Open University (Motzkau J. 'How Does Social Psychology Matter? Producing Knowledge—evaluating research', in Block 6 Online Commentary: The Production of Knowledge. The Open University; 2012). Our description of the modes is adapted from this material. To illustrate the use of the modes, an example is first outlined in the next subsection.

An example for critical evaluation

To illustrate the critical evaluation modes, explained later, we are going to use a genuine example from the literature. It relates to a paper published in the *BMJ* in 2010, at the height of the 2009–10 swine flu pandemic. The *BMJ* is a highly regarded international peer-reviewed medical journal with a high impact factor. According to its own website:

> *The journal has an impact factor of 17.4 (June 2015) and is ranked fifth among general medical journals. Its articles make news around the world on a daily basis and are routinely cited in clinical guidelines.*

The example we are using is a paper that concerned the safety and effectiveness of vaccines against the 2009–10 swine flu virus, an infection more officially known as H1N1 influenza, specifically when administered to children aged 12 years old and under. The full citation for the example paper, using the Vancouver style, is:

> *Waddington CS, Walker WT, Oeser C, Reiner A, John T, Wilkins S, et al. Safety and Immunogenicity of AS03B Adjuvanted Split Virion Versus Non-adjuvanted Whole Virion H1N1 Influenza Vaccine in UK Children Aged 6 Months–12 Years: Open Label, Randomised, Parallel Group, Multicentre Study. BMJ 2010;340:c2649. doi: 10.1136/ bmj.c2649.*

Recall a statement we made in Chapter 4 about journals such as the *BMJ*: 'The high impact factor of these journals generally tells us that they are respected publications, providing a certain level of guarantee that studies published within have been judged to be top-quality research. This is because high-impact journals receive more submissions and can therefore be more selective about the material they accept'. The reason we have selected a paper from the *BMJ* to discuss here is precisely to demonstrate that the publication source in itself does not inhibit an in-depth critical evaluation. If anything, the scientific method hinges on the critical evaluation of existing knowledge so that progress can be made. If Albert Einstein had not critiqued Isaac Newton's established theory of mechanics, he would not have developed the theory of relativity!

Before looking at the example paper, let us briefly consider the 2009–10 H1N1 influenza pandemic and the medical response. The pandemic emerged in 2009 and caused more than 280,000 deaths worldwide. At the time the World Health Organization (WHO) promoted an international vaccination plan that included the development, distribution, and administration of safe and effective vaccines against H1N1 influenza. The European Union licensure process was modified so that a new vaccine could be fast-tracked through the approval process, allowing GlaxoSmithKline to receive a marketing authorization for its mock-up vaccine developed in the pre-pandemic phase. After the H1N1 influenza virus was identified, the company made a variation to the product's composition strain, producing the vaccine Pandemrix (H1N1-AS03$_B$), an *adjuvanted* split-virion vaccine derived from egg culture. Baxter Vaccines also produced a *non-adjuvanted* whole-virion vaccine derived from Vero cell culture. The *BMJ* publication compared the safety and effectiveness of these two vaccines. A news report following the publication of the paper is presented in Box 7.2. Box 7.3 provides the scientific abstract from the original publication.

 Box 7.2   A news report published on the BBC News website in 2010

Child swine flu vaccine trial results published

A trial of swine flu vaccines given to children in Southampton and Oxford found they provided 'good protection' against the virus.

The Health Protection Agency conducted the study with the Universities of Bristol, Oxford, Southampton, Exeter, and St George's in London.

More than 900 children aged between six months and 12 years from the five cities were volunteered for the study.

Researchers said the children responded well and most side effects were minor. The trial compared two types of vaccine.

'Reassuring evidence'

Researchers said 98% of children under three responded well to two doses of the 'adjuvanted' vaccine, which contained immunity boosting agents.

The adjuvanted vaccine, also called the split virus vaccine, was the most commonly used on children during the pandemic but was also the most likely to cause side effects such as fever.

Only 80% of under threes responded to two doses of the 'whole virus' vaccine.

The difference between the vaccines in children over three was less pronounced, with 99% responding well to the adjuvanted version and 95% for the whole virus jab.

Dr Matthew Snape of the Oxford Vaccine Group at The University of Oxford said: 'Most children receiving either vaccine had no more than minor reactions, and this study provides reassuring evidence that both vaccines were well tolerated and likely to provide good protection against swine flu.'

He added: 'Traditionally the under threes don't tend to respond well to flu vaccines.

'This could show us the way to improve seasonal flu vaccines and help make a vaccine that generates a better response in young children.'

The study, published in the *British Medical Journal* today, is the first to be carried out comparing the immune response rates to the two vaccines in children aged between six months and 12 years.

Box 7.3   Full abstract of the 2010 *BMJ* publication

Abstract

Objectives To compare the safety, reactogenicity, and immunogenicity of an adjuvanted split virion H1N1 vaccine and a non-adjuvanted whole virion vaccine used in the pandemic immunisation programme in the United Kingdom.

Design Open label, randomised, parallel group, phase II study.

Setting Five UK centres (Oxford, Southampton, Bristol, Exeter, and London).

Participants Children aged 6 months to less than 13 years for whom a parent or guardian had provided written informed consent and who were able to comply with study procedures were eligible. Those with laboratory confirmed pandemic H1N1 influenza or clinically diagnosed disease meriting antiviral treatment, allergy to egg or any other vaccine components, or coagulation defects, or who were severely immunocompromised or had recently received blood products were excluded. Children were grouped by age: 6 months–<3 years (younger group) and 3–<13 years (older group). Recruitment was by media advertising and direct mailing. Recruitment visits were attended by 949 participants, of whom 943 were enrolled and 937 included in the per protocol analysis.

Interventions Participants were randomised 1:1 to receive AS03$_B$ (tocopherol based oil in water emulsion) adjuvanted split virion vaccine derived from egg culture or non-adjuvanted whole virion vaccine derived from cell culture. Both were given as two doses 21 days apart. Reactogenicity data were collected for one week after immunisation by diary card. Serum samples were collected at baseline and after the second dose.

Main outcome measures Primary reactogenicity end points were frequency and severity of fever, tenderness, swelling, and erythema after vaccination. Immunogenicity was measured by microneutralisation and haemagglutination inhibition assays. The primary immunogenicity objective was a comparison between vaccines of the percentage of participants showing seroconversion by the microneutralisation assay (fourfold rise to a titre of ≥1:40 from before vaccination to three weeks after the second dose).

Results Seroconversion rates were higher after the adjuvanted split virion vaccine than after the whole virion vaccine, most notably in the youngest children (163 of 166 participants with paired serum samples (98.2%, 95% confidence interval 94.8% to 99.6%) *v* 157 of 196 (80.1%, 73.8% to 85.5%), P<0.001) in children under 3 years and 226 of 228 (99.1%, 96.9% to 99.9%) *v* 95.9%, 92.4% to 98.1%, P=0.03) in those over 3 years) [sic]. The adjuvanted split virion vaccine was more reactogenic than the whole virion vaccine, with more frequent systemic reactions and severe local reactions in children aged over 5 years after dose one (13 (7.2%, 3.9% to 12%) *v* 2 (1.1%, 0.1% to 3.9%), P<0.001) and dose two (15 (8.5%, 4.8% to 13.7%) *v* 2 (1.1%, 0.1% to 4.1%), P<0.002) and after dose two in those under 5 years (15 (5.9%, 3.3% to 9.6%) *v* 0 (0.0%, 0% to 1.4%), P<0.001). Dose two of the adjuvanted split virion vaccine was more reactogenic than dose one, especially for fever ≥38°C in those aged under 5 (24 (8.9%, 5.8% to 12.9%) *v* 57 (22.4%, 17.5% to 28.1%), P<0.001).

Conclusions In this first direct comparison of an AS03$_B$ adjuvanted split virion versus whole virion non-adjuvanted H1N1 vaccine, the adjuvanted vaccine, while more reactogenic, was more immunogenic and, importantly, achieved high seroconversion rates in children aged less than 3 years. This indicates the potential for improved immunogenicity of influenza vaccines in this age group.

Trial registration Clinical trials.gov NCT00980850; ISRCTN89141709.

Applying the modes framework for macrolevel critical evaluation

As mentioned, different perspectives or modes can be adopted when evaluating, for example, a research study such as the one outlined earlier. Recall that these were described as *mode 1*: a within-perspective critique; *mode 2*: a-between perspective critique; and *mode 3*: a meta-perspective critique.

It is important at this stage to introduce one of the other concepts that you will become familiar with as a pharmacy student, namely 'evidence-based medicine', more broadly known as 'evidence-based practice'. A key component of evidence-based practice, covered in depth in Chapter 11, is the ability to read clinical papers in order to assess the weight of evidence being presented—essentially to decide whether or not the evidence should be used to guide patient care. As you will learn in Chapter 11, this assessment involves quality-rating the *conduct of the study*, as well as examining the *type of study* being presented (along an evidence hierarchy, e.g. whether the paper is a case study or a clinical trial). The current chapter extends beyond these aspects to also take into account the quality of *arguments*, the *basis and purpose of the research*, as well as the *wider impact of the publication*. These different levels of critique can be rationalized according to the mode model, which once understood can be applied selectively to your critical evaluation as needed.

Mode 1: a within-perspective critique

A *within-perspective* critique focuses on evaluating a study or paper according to the basic assumptions of the specific discipline. With the *BMJ* example publication we discussed a little earlier, we would ask, for example, whether, according to its own criteria (i.e. open-label, randomized, parallel-group, multicentre study), the study is appropriate and meets its aims. It might be appropriate to ask if the study was designed appropriately, whether the experiments were carried out accurately, or whether the data-collection tools were reliable. As we discuss in Chapter 11, a number of tools exist for evaluating the internal quality of different studies. Possible evaluative questions include whether any errors could have been made in participant selection; if there were problems with the type or number of participants recruited; and whether there might have been errors made in the way the data were collected or the study completed.

Another important point to consider at the within-perspective level is whether the study has real-world relevance—for example, whether it offers an important solution in the way the authors claim it does. This issue is known as ecological or external validity. At the core of this idea is an evaluation of the authors' claims about their findings, their interpretation of what the results mean, the robustness of the conclusions, whether these are plausible and valid, whether unproven claims are being made, and whether important issues have been overlooked.

It is important to say that mode 1 is not about engaging critically with the assumptions of the approach being taken. For example, here we are not criticizing the use of an open-label, randomized, parallel-group, multicentre study to examine the safety and effectiveness of the H1N1 vaccine. Instead, we are staying completely inside the perspective of the study. If, however, we were to criticize the concept of measuring vaccine safety through diary records or the use of an open-label, randomized study to examine it, then the evaluation moves into mode 2 or 3 critique. This is because we would be using those modes to challenge the basic assumptions of the original study.

Mode 2: a between-perspective critique

This mode involves the critic in assuming a completely different stance or position to that taken by the study authors when evaluating the study. It is easy to assume that the argument being presented by authors in the introduction of a paper, for example, is the only viable viewpoint; often, however, it is not. It is incredibly important to realize that what is written in the introduction of a paper has been put together specifically in order to justify the conduct of the study. However, this is no reason to accept that what is written is therefore *the only truth*.

For example, while an open-label, randomized, parallel-group, multicentre study might be one way of examining vaccine safety, another stance would be to use a multicentre case–control study to examine a causal link between the vaccine and a significant adverse effect. Or, for example, mode 2 would involve questioning the concept of vaccine safety as being measurable by adverse effects recordable within weeks of vaccine administration.

Mode 2, then, is about critically evaluating a study through the lens of another perspective. Here, the idea is to not take the written material at face value. Instead, you would step back and anchor yourself in another viewpoint. This is not a skill that comes naturally to many students, especially if they lack familiarity with other perspectives and approaches. The key is to ask questions about the text specifically in relation to other research methods or other perspectives that could have been adopted instead.

Mode 3: a meta-perspective critique

The meta-perspective mode involves stepping back from any specific perspective at all in order to evaluate the way the study or text you are reading is interpreting the evidence, defining the topic and contributing to knowledge. Think of this as a philosophical way of critiquing your reading material. As such, this mode involves thinking on a different level. What we are questioning within the meta-perspective mode is what the authors of your reading material are achieving by publishing their work at all—for example, in terms of the impact on people's ideas, influencing decisions, and giving credence to one viewpoint over another. In this perspective we are also interested in examining the historical context that allows one type of research or argument to arise, over another.

Specific questions to ask within this mode are around what concepts are being *taken for granted* in the written material: whether there are any hidden assumptions in the way a research question, for example, has been phrased; concepts defined; the study set up; the findings interpreted. Additional questions to ask are around what has not been included—for example, ideas not presented or asked about within the work, or population groups and individuals excluded from the work.

The main effort when evaluating within this mode is working out whether there are any problems as a result of the author(s)' approach—how does the particular way in which they have framed their work affect people, practices, decisions, behaviours, and so on? There could equally be beneficial effects from the research, to be explored at this level of critical evaluation. For example, the work might unearth a previously ignored or hidden area; it might benefit specific groups in the population, or add weight to a worthwhile but previously untested or contested hypothesis; it might empower better patient care, for example. In the context of the *BMJ* example paper, we might specifically ask about who funded the research in the first place, whether the authors declared any conflicts of interest, and whether there were other vaccines available that could also have been tested (but were not).

Finally, the meta-perspective mode encourages consideration of the historical context within which the research takes place. A key question to ask in this mode is how the research or paper you are evaluating reflects the ideas of the time and place it was conducted or written in; are there specific ethical, cultural, political issues of the time, for example, influencing the way the findings have been interpreted or debated? You would also be interested in knowing whether the paper reflects the experiences or concerns of specific groups or generalizable populations; whether the work is focused in one particular country or context, or whether it addresses an international agenda.

Another way of thinking about this is to consider what the written material might have looked like if it was put together 20 years earlier, or, indeed, now, for an older publication. Would the same questions have been asked, the same arguments put forward; if not, why not? What does the paper add to current knowledge; how does it help answer questions that are relevant to the here and now? Does the material acknowledge its own limitations in terms of historical context? With our specific examples, you might ask therefore what new knowledge we now have about the H1N1 vaccine that would invalidate the findings of the *BMJ* example publication.

Critical evaluation of the example paper: one standpoint

We are going to ask a series of questions (which span the three modes) as we conduct a critical evaluation of the *BMJ* example paper, namely:

1. What is the main argument presented by this paper?
2. Are the authors experts in their field? Do they have a biased agenda or perspective?
3. Is the text up to date?
4. Is the evidence being presented to support the main argument convincing?
5. Is there a fair and balanced viewpoint being put forward; have the authors presented evidence to support alternative views?
6. Are the conclusions reasonable based on the findings and other evidence?

Looking at the *BMJ* example paper, and noting that the title is 'Safety and Immunogenicity of $AS03_B$ Adjuvanted Split Virion Versus Non-adjuvanted Whole Virion H1N1 Influenza Vaccine...', we will focus on aspects relating to assessment of the 'safety' of the vaccine and ideas around adjuvanted vaccines. The study reported on vaccine safety and how children reacted to the vaccine by asking parents/guardians to use diary cards to record temperature, injection-site reactions, systemic symptoms, and medications given. In addition, medically important adverse events (judged as ongoing solicited reactions or events necessitating a doctor's visit or study withdrawal after day seven of vaccination) were also recorded on a diary card. The authors stated that all data from case report forms and participant diary cards were double-entered and verified on a computer. It seems clear, then, that the paper has framed the collection of safety data in one particular way, through recording symptoms and reactions in the weeks following the vaccine.

Using a meta-perspective mode of critical evaluation, we are going to examine the historical context within which the work in the *BMJ* example paper was conducted. We are going to look, in particular, at the reporting of the safety outcome. Based on their findings, the authors begin the discussion section: 'In this head to head study of an adjuvanted split virion H1N1 pandemic vaccine and a non-adjuvanted whole virion vaccine in children, both vaccines were well tolerated.' Note the statement about the vaccines being well tolerated. An adjuvant is a vaccine component that speeds up the desired immune response to a vaccine by working with the vaccine. In fact, it became necessary to use adjuvants in the 2009–10 pandemic as researchers saw a poor immune response to the pre-pandemic vaccine; subsequently, the WHO encouraged the use of adjuvants as a way of making best use of sparse supplies of the antigen (a molecule capable of inducing an immune response). Sadly, however, since the publication of the *BMJ* example paper and the mass vaccination programme (about 30 million doses of the AS03 adjuvanted vaccine were given during the pandemic) the H1N1 AS03 vaccine has been scientifically linked with an increased incidence of childhood-onset cases of narcolepsy.

Within a meta-perspective critical evaluation mode, then, it becomes possible to see that, at the time the *BMJ* study was conducted, it would have been reasonable to frame a safety investigation as a short-term endeavour—because the data on narcolepsy have only come to light through the real-life experience with 30 million doses of the AS03 adjuvanted vaccine.

The question of why the AS03 adjuvanted vaccine was investigated in a small study recruiting fewer than 1000 patients is an important one. It has also been noted that while there had been very little clinical experience with the AS03 adjuvant in 2009–10, an alternative adjuvant (MF59) had been used in seasonal influenza vaccines since 1997, with more than 45 million doses having been distributed, but it raised no substantial safety concerns. Interestingly, since 2009, no association has been found between the H1N1 MF59 vaccine and narcolepsy.

Moving back to the within-perspective mode 1, we could critically ask why the *BMJ* example study recruited a sample of 949 participants. Crossing to the between-perspective mode 2, we would ask whether an open-label, randomized, parallel-group, multicentre study was really the right approach to assessing certainly the safety of the H1N1 AS03 vaccine. We would assert that the study design was, in fact, flawed in light of the minimal existing experience with the AS03 adjuvant at the time.

Moving again to the meta-perspective mode, we would question who, in fact, paid for the study to examine the safety of the H1N1 AS03 vaccine in this way, whether the manufacturer GlaxoSmithKline was involved, and whether the authors declared a conflict of interest in relation to existing relationships with the company. If you think that this is nearing a conspiracy theory, it might interest you to know that the month after the publication of the *BMJ* example paper we have been discussing, the *BMJ* also published a piece on the pandemic entitled 'Conflicts of Interest. WHO and the Pandemic Flu "Conspiracies"'. The article is introduced as follows: 'Key scientists advising the World Health Organization on planning for an influenza pandemic had done paid work for pharmaceutical firms that stood to gain from the guidance they were preparing.'

Within the meta-perspective mode of critical evaluation, it would be important to acknowledge that the drug company, GlaxoSmithKline, could gain a lot from the way in which the *BMJ* example publication framed its findings in favour of the vaccine. Although the study was not funded by vaccine manufacturers, some of the study authors declared having received research grants and honoraria from vaccine manufacturers, having participated in advisory boards for such companies, or having received financial assistance from such companies to attend conferences in the past. This potential conflict of interest may have affected the way in which the findings were framed and vaccine safety subsequently discussed, including in the media—for example, by choosing not to mention the limited experience with the AS03 adjuvant and known or hypothesized problems with adjuvants. It might help you to return to the BBC News report of the paper, shown in Box 7.2, specifically: 'Researchers said the children responded well and most side effects were minor.' Although this is not definitive proof of any wrongdoing, it does, nonetheless, bring into question the potential for undue influence to have affected the communication around the research findings.

We might form a conclusion that, in fact, the *BMJ* example paper was limited in its scope, despite being useful at the time in terms of providing reassurance about the more immediate side effects of the H1N1 AS03 vaccine; it did not examine the long-term safety of the vaccine (it was not designed to) and did not compare safety with an existing adjuvanted vaccine, known to have a better side - effect profile. Returning to the historical context, as we now know that the H1N1 AS03 vaccine is associated with a higher incidence of narcolepsy, the *BMJ* example paper is, in fact, no longer relevant in terms of one of its original aims, which was to provide assurances about the safety of this vaccine.

How to write with a critical voice

Having outlined our own critical evaluation of the *BMJ* example paper, we have already illustrated writing with a critical voice through an example. In this section, we are going to provide a brief framework to help you construct your own critical evaluation of material. Where appropriate, we will refer back to the critical evaluation of the *BMJ* example paper. What we do not wish to do here is extensively repeat the guidance we have already provided in Chapter 5, relating to the writing of essays and the use of the framework 'point–evidence–explanation' to structure your writing. We would suggest that you should read Chapter 5 (if you have not already done so) before returning to the current section.

Recall, then, that the framework 'point–evidence–explanation' can be a useful way of demonstrating your argument. To summarize, the element 'point' is about writing clearly what you are arguing for; 'evidence' is the existing material you are drawing on to make your particular claim; and 'explanation' is then your logical reasoning for why the particular evidence you have cited supports your claim. Some people also advocate incorporating a 'qualification' element, which is a way of acknowledging the weaknesses of your evidence in fully supporting your claim. For example, with our critique of the *BMJ* example paper, we use the following qualification: 'Although this is not definitive proof of any wrongdoing....'

Box 7.4   An example of a *flawed* argument.

Point: The H1N1-AS03 vaccine is safe to use in children.

Evidence: A *BMJ* paper published in 2010 examined the safety of the vaccine in children and showed that most side effects were minor.

Explanation: The *BMJ* paper demonstrates the safety of the vaccine when used in children. Therefore, I would endorse the use of this vaccine should another H1N1 pandemic arise.

Qualifications: If a new H1N1 pandemic came about, a newer vaccine would have to be produced using antigen specific to the new strain.

It is sometimes useful to read a bad example in order to learn what a good example would look like. We have used a bad example to illustrate our point in Box 7.4. Note that the example is a caricatured and flawed extension of what we have been discussing in relation to the *BMJ* example paper.

As we stated in the previous paragraph, the example in Box 7.4 is purposefully a flawed argument. As we know, there is a *BMJ* publication that claims H1N1 AS03 vaccine is safe. However, as we have been examining in this chapter, there is newer information to suggest that the AS03 adjuvant is linked to a higher incidence of narcolepsy. The fact that the *BMJ* study exists does not prove that the vaccine is safe to use in children. To make the claim in Box 7.4 would be to ignore other existing evidence and simply present one version of the truth. This would make the argument and the explanation provided imbalanced because the writing has not adequately explored other evidence when supporting the claim.

If you wanted to write a good critical argument, you would ask yourself questions such as: what other existing evidence contributes to our knowledge about the safety of the H1N1 AS03 vaccine; what is the relative weight of the different pieces of evidence in this field? You would also have to convey through your writing the significance of the argument, the relevance of the evidence, and, importantly, the strength of the conclusions.

As well as making sure that your argument is sound and balanced, you can use certain tools to help you convey the logic and progress of your argument. Recall that in Chapter 5, for example, we talked about focusing each paragraph on one particular point, and also using signposting at the end of a paragraph to indicate the topic of the next. We also looked at examples of linking words and their use. Ultimately, you will need to structure your writing to make a clear argument, identifying the claims you make, the relevant evidence, and the justification for your conclusions. To do this, you have to show how you have analysed and evaluated the material in a balanced way. In addition to that you have to take clear strides forward in your reasoning, while showing how the different parts fit together to make an interconnected piece.

As we hope you can see, we have tried in our own critical evaluation of the *BMJ* example paper to focus each paragraph on one particular point:

- the first focuses on introducing the concept of safety as a focus of the paper;
- the second examines more closely the way safety data were collected;

- the third drills down further to question the study design in light of a lack of experience with the AS03 adjuvanted vaccine;
- the fourth examines the potential for vaccine manufacturers to have exerted undue influence around communication of the research findings;
- the final paragraph brings matters to a close by highlighting that the study has been superseded by new findings.

We have also used ample linking words such as:

- in addition to that; also; it seems clear then; in fact;
- subsequently; although; then; because;
- it has also been noted that; while; interestingly;
- we would assert; moving again; it might interest you to know;
- it would be important to acknowledge; for example;
- it might help you to know; nonetheless; we might form a conclusion.

Feel free to examine the text for additional linking words.

An additional device is to add context and examples, not only in the introduction to your work, but also in the main body, where needed. For example, you might give a description of a theory or concept, such as drug–receptor interactions, or drug excretion, or you might give a historical account of a situation, such as the past treatment of non-small-cell lung cancer. Look back at our critical evaluation and notice how we have added context and examples in several places. For example, 'An adjuvant is a vaccine component that speeds up the desired immune response to a vaccine by working with the vaccine', and 'WHO encouraged the use of adjuvants as a way of making best use of sparse supplies of antigen (a molecule capable of inducing an immune response)'.

 Key points

- Your degree will involve you acquiring knowledge, comprehending information, applying your knowledge, analysing, synthesizing, and evaluating.
- You can apply critical thinking to almost anything you read while studying for your degree.
- Critical thinking is the objective analysis and evaluation of an issue in order to form a judgement.
- To read effectively, initially scan and skim the text to judge its relevance before actively engaging to understand the material.
- To critically evaluate you will need to question the validity of the information you read, the arguments made, the evidence presented, and the conclusions reached.
- To think critically you can explore the similarities and differences of what you read compared with other published work.
- You can use the three 'modes' to frame your critical evaluation: a within-perspective, a between-perspective, and a meta-perspective mode.

- When critiquing a paper in a within-perspective mode, you would be asking whether the material you are reading is appropriate and meets its aims, according to its own criteria.

- When critiquing a paper in a between-perspective mode, assume a different stance to that taken by the study authors, and ask if another perspective would have yielded different arguments.

- When critiquing a paper in a meta-perspective mode, critique the philosophy of your reading material, specifically by asking who gains from the arguments made and whether there are historical influences on what has been written.

- When writing with a critical voice use the 'point–evidence–explanation' framework to structure your writing, qualifying evidence that is weaker in its nature.

- Devote one paragraph to each particular point, and use linking words to produce a well-connected and laid-out argument.

- Add examples and context to your critical writing where relevant.

 Further reading

Critical Appraisal Skills Programme (CASP): http://www.casp-uk.net

The equator network: Enhancing the QUAlity and Transparency Of health Research: http://www.equator-network.org/reporting-guidelines

Mayfield Handbook of Technical & Scientific Writing: http://www.mhhe.com/mayfieldpub/tsw/home.htm

8 Preparing for and sitting exams

 ## Overview

Some people can find preparing for and sitting exams a particularly stressful period of academic life. At this stage of your learning, you may think that you are already very familiar with the exam process and the different types of assessment. Indeed, you will have probably been exposed to different types of assessment in order to get to where you are now. What you may not have been aware of, however, is the variability in exam formats. An awareness of these different formats, as well as being ready to set yourself enough time for revision as you prepare for exams, and knowing how to cope with stress and panic, can potentially improve your exam experience and ultimately your grades.

In an ideal world, learning should not be led by assessment –you shouldn't be learning purely to pass exams—so it's best to avoid getting into this mindset where possible. After all, once you graduate you are expected to undertake some form of continual education to keep up to date with professional practice, without the need for assessment. This chapter will give you an awareness of the different exam question formats you may come across and how best to prepare for and sit exams.

 ## Learning outcomes

You should be able to demonstrate knowledge and understanding of the following after working through this chapter:

- different question formats used in written exam papers;
- creation of an effective revision timetable;
- tips and hints in dealing with stress and sitting the exam paper.

Exam question formats

When you think about exams, you may automatically think about multiple-choice questions (MCQs), and short- and long-answer/essay questions. In most cases you will be correct in your thinking. Up to now you will probably have experienced closed-book exams in which you have no access to any reference material and hence you rely totally on memory recall. In a university context, however, you may experience a mixture of both open- and closed-book exams, with the 'open book' meaning that you are allowed to use certain reference material. Whichever is the case, it is useful to have an awareness of the types of questions you may be presented with and what they intend to test. Table 8.1 provides you with some exam question formats you may come across. For the purpose of this chapter we will focus mainly on traditional written exam papers, which may include MCQ and/or short- or long-answer questions.

Table 8.1 Exam question formats

Format of exam question	What is this question type trying to test?
Oral: questions are delivered and answered face-to-face	In most cases, the purpose of an oral exam will be to assess your understanding of the subject area, your ability to articulate your ideas, and explain your thought processes, and so on
Practical	Practical exams examine your ability to perform specific tasks. They look at whether you are able to *apply* your knowledge/understanding of a subject as opposed to just regurgitating factual information. There is usually a problem-solving element or a requirement to perform a specific task, e.g. measuring volumes, extemporaneous dispensing, or preparing a labelled medicinal product
Problem-solving	Requires you to have a thorough understanding of the subject area in order to solve a problem or derive a solution. Usually, this type of question relies on solving a series of steps to get to the final answer, which may include solving equations or pharmaceutical calculations. Similar to practical exams, these questions are seeking to test your ability to apply knowledge
Multiple-choice questions (MCQs)	Typically, MCQs require you to choose a correct answer to a question from a range of possible answers that are given to you. There are many formats to this type of question, which will be discussed later on. However, the main purpose of MCQs is to test the depth and breadth of your factual knowledge
Short answer	Can vary from being questions that require one-word answers to those requiring answers that are a paragraph or two in length. They are mainly intended to test your ability to recall specific information (similar to MCQs), but may also require some interpretation or application of these facts
Long answer/essays	These questions come in various formats and usually involve the words 'describe', 'discuss', and 'explain'. They encourage you to read widely so that you are more knowledgeable about your subject as a whole, and are designed to test the depth of your understanding of a subject area, as well as the ability to express your ideas in written form

Multiple choice questions

MCQs come in different formats, ranging from simple to assertion reason types, all testing students' factual knowledge of a broad range of content with some testing to a higher level of cognition. They are typically composed of one question with multiple possible answers, including the correct answer and several incorrect answers.

Simple MCQs

The simplest types of MCQs are true/false or questions for which you select one correct answer, which rely on memory recall (or guesswork!). As their name implies, questions in a true/false style require you to indicate whether a particular statement is true or false. There is a 50% chance of getting the right answer, so these types of MCQs are not used as much to test knowledge of a broad range of content. True/false-type questions have begun to fall out of use as there is much evidence in the medical literature showing that these questions are poor discriminators of knowledge and understanding.

Example 1

Consider the following statements. Indicate whether they are true or false.

1. Insulin is important in the regulation of blood glucose levels (True/False).
2. Aspirin has antiplatelet activity (True/False).
3. A cough suppressant is the best recommendation for treating a chesty cough (True/False).

An example of a one-correct-answer question is as follows:

Example 2

To be **legally** valid, a written prescription for a prescription-only veterinary medicine (POM-V) must include which **ONE** of the following?

A. The professional qualifications of the prescriber.

B. The words 'for animal treatment only'.

C. The weight of the animal for which the medicine is prescribed.

D. The indication for the medicine.

E. The words 'do not exceed the stated dose'.

This type of MCQ is one of the most commonly used and is easy to answer if you have re-vised the material. You will usually know straight away if you know the answer, but it's always useful to read the question and look at the answers a couple of times to confirm your initial thoughts. As with any of the MCQs described here, you may decide to guess the answer if you don't know it, thinking there is a 20–25% (if 5 or 4 options are available, respectively) chance of getting it right. This might be more beneficial than leaving the answer box blank, but be aware that if there is negative marking involved (i.e. marks will be deducted for incorrect answers), then it is best not to guess.

You may also see what is referred to as single-*best*-answer questions. ('Best' or 'most likely' are common phrases used.) This type of MCQ provides you with a list of options which all could be true (or are not completely wrong), but requires you to choose what you think is the *best*. These types of MCQs are quite challenging as they require you to think more deeply about the question, rationalizing the information to get the most appropriate answer.

Example 3

A 50-year-old woman has been managing her diabetes by only controlling her diet. She has a friend who has been managed on antidiabetic tablets, which seems to have helped reduce her blood sugar more effectively. The patient finds it quite difficult to manage her diet and wonders if taking an antidiabetic drug will give her better control of her diabetes. You assess her diet and this seems fine, but her blood sugar levels are still higher than expected. The patient is also obese. What would be the best choice of drug for this patient?

A. Insulin.

B. Gliclazide.

C. Metformin.

D. Acarbose.

E. Sitagliptin.

In this example, you would need to know about the stepwise management of diabetes, and look at any information given to you that would confirm or rule out the use of a particular drug. Here you are required not to regurgitate factual knowledge, but to use that knowledge and apply it to that scenario. So the best answer would be metformin because it is used as a first-line medication and is recommended for use in patients who are obese. Insulin does not fit the patient profile, gliclazide can cause weight gain so is not good for obese patients, acarbose is not recommended as a first-line medication, and sitagliptin could be used but only if the patient cannot tolerate metformin.

Multiple response questions

Multiple response questions (MRQs) require more thought than simple MCQs, and usually involve multiple true/false-type questions. Students can select more than one answer, and more than one of the possible answers given can be correct. This means that a MRQ with four alternatives can be answered in 16 different ways. MRQs are normally more difficult to answer than simple MCQs because you need to consider simultaneously more information, a bit like the single-best-answer question described in the previous subsection.

Example 4

Consider the following question:

A 50-year-old woman has been managing her diabetes by only controlling her diet. She has a friend who has been managed on metformin, which seems to have helped reduce her blood sugar more effectively. The patient finds it quite difficult to manage her diet and wonders whether taking metformin will give her better control of her diabetes. In relation to this case, indicate whether each statement is true or false.

A. She should be told that metformin is a possible option for her.

B. The problems associated with metformin should be discussed with her.

C. She could be put on insulin instead of metformin.

D. She should be advised that further treatment is not required.

E. You should find out more about her control of diet.

Like the single-best-answer question example (Example 3), you would be required to look carefully at all the options and relate them to what you know about the topic.

Alternatively, you may be presented with the following type of multiple-response MCQ, which is the most commonly used format of this type.

> ONE or MORE of the responses is (are) correct. Decide which of the responses is (are) correct. Then choose:
>
> A. If 1, 2, and 3 are correct.
> B. If 1 and 2 only are correct.
> C. If 2 and 3 only are correct.
> D. If 1 only is correct.
> E. If 3 only is correct.

Example 5

Consider the following question:

Which of the following is/are **legal** requirement(s) for a registered pharmacy? The premises must:

1. Hold a contract to dispense NHS prescriptions.
2. Close during the absence of the Responsible Pharmacist.
3. Have specific standard operating procedures in place.

This type of MCQ can be confusing to answer at first because only one option could be correct, or all three could be correct (or, indeed, somewhere in between). If you are certain about what is/are correct, then looking carefully at the options for A–E will usually help you get to the answer.

For Example 5, if you were certain only option 3 was correct then the answer would be E. However, if you thought that options 1 and 3 were correct and option 2 was definitely wrong, then you would need to think again, because there is no 'if 1 and 3 only are correct' option, so you would be left with D or E as the answer. At this point you will have more certainty about your answer.

Matching items

Matching-item questions are another more complex version of simple MCQs. They require in-depth knowledge and reasoning, and an understanding of several aspects of a topic.

The most commonly used type of matching question is the extended matching question, which uses multiple questions and answers based on a common theme. Extended matching questions typically use vignettes, or scenarios, to which you have to match the answer. They introduce an element of problem solving into the question. These types of questions are commonly used in the pre-registration exam.

Example 6

Consider the following question:

A. Morphine sulphate injection.

B. Diclofenac tablets.

C. Ibuprofen liquid.

D. Oxycodone tablets.

E. Paracetamol liquid.

F. Aspirin dispersible tablets.

G. Pethidine tablets.

H. Co-codamol tablets.

For the patients described below, select the most suitable analgesic from the list. Each option may be used once, more than once, or not at all.
A 7-year-old boy who suffers from asthma has developed a high fever, as well as a runny nose. The boy has no known allergies and hasn't taken analgesics before.
A 50-year-old woman has chronic pain from bone cancer. She has completed her course of chemotherapy and is now under palliative care. She has allergies to morphine salts. She has been using tramadol at the maximum recommended dose, but this is no longer controlling her pain.

As you can probably tell from looking at the examples, these require a lot more effort to answer, and a lot more time to get to the right answer. Multiple diseases are presented so it's not only a matter of knowing about the drugs, but also what would be the best, and safest for the patient described. If it helps, underline keywords or sentences. As it is more difficult to guess the answer to this type of question, it is a truer test of your knowledge than the previous MCQ types described.

Assertion-reason questions

Assertion-reason questions are used to explore cause and effect, and to identify relationships between statements. Hence, they test the application of knowledge/analysis of a problem. A typical representation of this is as follows:

Directions summarized

	First statement	Second statement	
A	True	True	Second statement is *a correct explanation* of the first
B	True	True	Second statement is NOT *a correct explanation* of the first
C	True	False	
D	False	True	
E	False	False	

Example 7

Consider the following question:

Statement 1	Statement 2
An entry needs to be made in the Controlled Drugs (CD) Register for patient-returned Schedule 2 controlled drugs.	It is a legal requirement for patient-returned Schedule 2 controlled drugs to be destroyed in the presence of an authorized witness.

These can be quite challenging, particularly when answers to statements A and B are true, as they require additional thought to explore cause and effect. A useful tip to help you determine whether the first and second statements are related is to introduce the word 'because' in between both statements: is the first statement true *because* of the second statement being true?

Short-answer questions

Short-answer questions are most often used to test basic knowledge of key facts and terms, but can also be used to test higher thinking skills, including analysis or evaluation. Compared with MCQs these types of questions make it more difficult for you to guess the answer. However, they do provide you with more opportunity to explain and show your understanding.

Example 8

You are working in a pharmacy and assume the role of the responsible pharmacist. You decide to go out for lunch, leaving the pharmacy without a pharmacist. While away on lunch, a customer comes into the pharmacy to collect their dispensed prescription. Is your dispenser allowed to give out the prescription? Justify your answer.

In Example 8, it is not sufficient to answer 'yes' or 'no', and you will be required to justify your answer by writing a few sentences with reasoning for saying 'yes' or 'no'. Always ensure that if the question asks for you to 'explain', 'justify', 'provide with examples', 'illustrate', and so on, that you actually do so, as a simple answer with no corroborating evidence of understanding will not give you full marks. Also be mindful of how many marks the short-answer question is worth as it is unlikely that you will need to write more than one or two paragraphs of text for a 5-mark question, for example. Also, the amount of space given to write your answer can sometimes guide you as to how much detail is required.

Remember that the examiner will be expecting you to relay discrete pieces of information relevant to the question, so don't try and write down everything you know about the subject as this will be a waste of your exam time and won't gain you any extra marks.

Long-answer questions/essays

Essay questions require written responses, which can vary in length from a couple of paragraphs to many pages. Like short-answer questions, they provide you with an opportunity to explain your understanding and show how you can apply your knowledge. However, essays make it harder for you to bluff your way through an answer as they are less structured than short-answer questions. We discuss essay writing in more detail in Chapter 5.

Oral examinations

Oral exams allow students to respond directly to questions and/or to present prepared statements, and can typically take at least 10–15 minutes per 'exam station', although the actual length can depend on what is being assessed. Sometimes oral exams are referred to as a viva voce ('viva', for short), which means 'by word of mouth'. You may encounter 'vivas' when defending your project dissertation, for example.

Another situation where you are most likely to encounter an oral exam is during objective structured clinical examinations (OSCEs), where you may be asked to respond to a patient's symptoms by asking relevant questions, to provide drug counselling, or to take a drug history. This latter type of oral exam is now becoming more popular within health care courses because it allows you to demonstrate the application of your knowledge and skills, as opposed to essays or MCQs, which only demonstrate that you know the information.

Finally, you may encounter assessment of oral presentations, and sometimes poster presentations, where your ability to explain a particular topic, assignment, project, and so on, in a clear, logical, and reasoned way is tested. Usually this is followed up by having to answer questions about your presentation or poster, which further verifies your understanding of the work undertaken.

We discuss a range of verbal assessments, including vivas and OSCEs, in more detail in Chapter 6.

Revision planning and time management

It is easy to underestimate how much time you need to revise and prepare for exams. You may feel that there is a lot of material to cover but not enough time to do it all. More often than not, revision is left until the last minute, with a culture of 'question spotting' (a process of trying to guess or predict certain topics that will come up in the exam and only revising these topics) then becoming the norm. Question spotting is highly discouraged and it is extremely important not to leave revision until the last minute. You can use various strategies to help prepare for exams, some of which will be outlined in the following subsections. You may already be aware of many of these strategies, but it is surprising how much information is overlooked, not apparent, or is forgotten about.

We will consider planning and time management under five themes: timetabling, the environment, use of study techniques, mental preparation, and pre-exam checklist.

Timetabling

Setting out a timetable for your study is one of the simplest things to do. You should know when the exam period is. Once you know your exam dates, write these down and then organize your revision accordingly. You may want to give some exams more preparation time than others, so think about how much time you will need to prepare for each exam, and

(a) Week number	Monday	Tuesday	Wednesday	Thursday	Friday	Saturday	Sunday
1	Module 1 Pharmaceutics Module 2 Pharmacology	Module 3 Physiology Module 4 Practice	Modules 1 and 2	Modules 3 and 4	Modules 1 and 2 Study group	Day off	Modules 3 and 4
2	Day off	Module 1	Module 2	Module 3	Module 4	Job	Module 1
3							
4							
5							
6							
7							

(b)	Monday	Tuesday	Wednesday	Thursday	Friday	Saturday	Sunday
Morning	Module 1 revision	Module 3 revision	Gym	Module 3 revision	Module 1 revision	Day off	Module 3 revision
Afternoon	Module 2 revision	Module 4 revision	Module 1 revision	Module 4 revision	Study group		Module 4 revision
Evening	Gym	Job	Module 2 revision	Job	Module 2 revision		Night off

Figure 8.1 Part examples of (a) long-term and (b) weekly revision timetables.

which ones might need more time than others. Examples of revision timetables are shown in Figure 8.1. It is worth noting that these are examples and the number of weeks of revision required will vary depending on the assessments being undertaken (some may need more, some less time).

When planning what you will revise and how much time you need to spend on a particular topic, it helps if you ask yourself the following questions:

- Do I have all the material I need (lecture notes, practical reports, workshop material)?
- What are the most important topics? Be careful not to only focus on these.
- Which topics do I know the best and can probably spend the least time on?
- Which topics do I need most support with? These will probably need more revision time.
- Which topics are compulsory to know?
- What kinds of questions will there be in the exam? Is there a choice of question?

Once you have considered all these questions then think carefully about how you will fit this all in to the time available to you. There will inevitably be times when you find yourself not working according to plan because you think you have enough time (poor time management), or you are feeling overwhelmed, or are a perfectionist, or just bored. So how can you help yourself to stick to your plan? You may want to think about setting small goals, having regular breaks, or planning other activities that are part of your daily routine. When making a revision plan also factor in time for sleep, breaks, meals, and attendance at university for tutorials, and so on. If you have a part-time job outside the university you should consider either giving this up or at least taking a break from it to leave yourself more time to concentrate on your studies. The same applies if you have family commitments, such as child care or looking after elderly relatives; could someone else undertake these duties until after your exams?

Also, make sure you allow some flexibility within your plan: having it planned to the second can create stress and anxiety, especially if you don't stick to plan or some other crisis occurs. In other words, always try and prepare for the unexpected, and be realistic about how much time you can actually spend on revision. Aiming for an 18-hour day may not always be productive, and so you need to figure out how much you can feasibly do. Try and break the day up as much as possible and involve some relaxation time and rest to help you feel less stressed and so more likely to stick to your timetable. You may find that revising in blocks of 2 or 3 hours with small breaks works for you. In addition, not spending the whole day on one module or topic but alternating modules or topics every few hours will keep you more motivated and will allow you to cover a wider range of material. It may also avoid the panic that comes with running out of time and not having covered anything on a particular module. Finally, remember to monitor your progress against your revision plan, so that the time you spend on different topics meets your needs.

The environment

The space you work in can make a difference to how well you study and how well you stick to your plan. Making your environment as study friendly as possible reduces the chance of any distractions, mental fatigue, or discomfort from occurring. Think about the following questions:

- Do I have enough space to work in (non-cluttered, ability to spread out)?
- Do I have enough light to be able to read clearly and not strain my eyes?
- Is my work area too hot or too cold?
- Do I have any distractions in my work space (television, radio, games consoles, bed, family demands)? Some people work well in a quiet room, whereas others concentrate better if there is some background noise. Also working on your bed is not really conducive to preparing your mind for studying!
- Do I have an area where I can relax?

Think about what works for you and make sure you stick to it.

Study techniques

You may have already done an exercise that looks at what type of learning style you have. Are you a visual learner who prefers using pictures and images? Do you prefer sound and music, or are you a social learner who prefers to learn in groups or with other people, or do you prefer to work alone? Whatever your style, when it comes to revision, you need to make a real effort to understand what you are learning, rather than just memorizing information. The memorization of facts does not allow you to think around problems and you are likely to forget the information more quickly. To ensure you understand the material you learn, it might be useful to think about the following:

- Can you identify common themes within topics?
- Is the information related to other topics in any way?
- Does knowing how to solve one problem help with solving other problems?
- Can you apply a mind map or spider diagram to your topics?

A common revision technique is to use visual aids. Typically this involves condensing all the information you have learnt into a one-page diagram. An example is given for hyperglycaemia (high blood glucose characteristic in diabetes) in Figure 8.2. You could also use spider diagrams, which help summarize and connect ideas about a topic (Figure 8.3). Mind maps are also a form of visual aid, which are covered in Chapter 2. The use of visual aids helps you to recall the information quickly when you next revisit the topic during your revision.

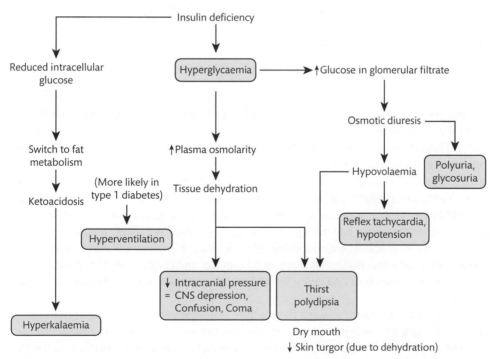

Figure 8.2 Example of a visual aid to remember the complications and symptoms associated with high blood glucose (hyperglycaemia).

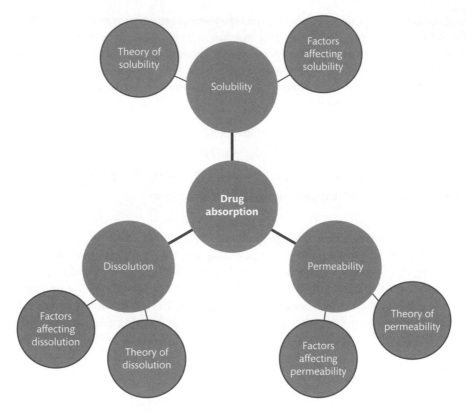

Figure 8.3 Example of a spider diagram.

If you are a social learner then speaking to other people or studying in groups may be use-ful for you. Sometimes, just explaining an answer to a question to a layperson (not a fellow student) helps to ensure you are able to explain things in a clear and concise manner. Getting together with friends to answer 'mock questions' (or even writing your own 'mock questions') can also be a useful exercise as you are able to discuss your answers and get different perspec-tives on what the question is asking and what the answer would be. However, particular care is needed when writing your own questions because the assumption would be that whoever created the model answer had the right answer(s), which may not always be the case. It is best to get the answer checked by a tutor before disseminating it to the rest of the group. Having a debate with your fellow students is also a useful exercise, and can be one of the most effective ways to challenge yourself *and* revise, as long as you make sure you all stay focused on the topic at hand.

Some people also like to re-write their lecture notes (summarizing as bullet points or as tables, or using index cards), which can be effective, but also very time consuming.

Memory aids can also be used, which usually involves a 'trigger word' that is linked with a particular topic. Creating mnemonics is commonly done to help recall larger pieces of infor-mation. Mnemonics are usually a word, phrase, or formula created to learn facts, which can easily be remembered. For example, a common mnemonic used in pharmacy for responding to symptoms is WWHAM:

Who is it for?

What are the symptoms?

How long have they had it?

Anything tried already?

Medication being taken?

Looking at past or sample (mock) papers and practising the questions is the most obvious way of preparing for exams. This helps you get used to the format of the questions, and the different sections of the paper, and also to plan how long you may need to spend on each section. One of the best ways to make use of past papers is to simulate exam conditions by not having your notes at hand and undertaking the exercise in the time allotted for the actual exam (for a closed-book exam). For an open-book exam you may want to find out what texts or notes you are allowed to take into the exam or will be provided, consider getting familiar with the text or notes that you will need, and making sure that the notes you prepare for your exams are concise, easily understood, and easily accessed. (Preparing a folder is a useful way to do this.) When writing a practice answer to a question, however, be realistic: it is unlikely anybody will write a perfect answer in the real exam.

More recently, study and/or revision apps, including YouTube videos, have become widespread and offer portability, user friendliness, and a more fun way of preparing for exams. Various apps are available, which allow you to prepare your own flash cards (video, voice, or text formats), provide tips for revision, create your own quizzes and MCQs, create mind maps, and create revision plans. A quick browse through Android- or Apple-based app sites reveals many aids for revision—some free, some requiring a fee to be paid. Although technically not a revision app, the Royal Pharmaceutical Society has developed an app, *RPharmS-iRx*, which is designed for undergraduate and postgraduate health care professionals to help develop their knowledge and understanding of using medicines safely and effectively. In terms of video-based tutorials, the Khan Academy is one of the more well-known educational support providers and offers free access to tutorials covering a wide range of topics.

In any event, whichever type of learner you are or whichever revision technique you use, knowing what works best for you is very important.

Mental preparation

Motivation is one of the biggest issues for revision. There are various strategies you can adopt to help maintain motivation. These include taking regular breaks, starting with topics that interest you or are easier to study, and planning rewards for when you achieve your goals.

Taking regular breaks is quite important. As mentioned previously, there is no point in working 18 hours a day if the quality of your revision is poor. In fact, studying for long periods without a break can be counterproductive because the amount of knowledge you can retain over a particular period of time is generally limited. The optimal length of study time varies from person to person: you may find that 2 hours is your limit, after which nothing 'sinks in'

Box 8.1 Pre-examination checklist

- Double-check the date, time, and place of your exam.
- Double-check how long the exam will be.
- Plan your route and journey time (check there are no scheduled disruptions, strikes, or maintenance work on roads or rail). At least a few hours before your exam, double-check your route and make sure you add some extra time for any unforeseen issues.
- Make sure you know the examination rules and what stationery you are allowed to take into the exam. (For example, if it is an open-book exam, check the resources you are allowed to take in. More generally, check whether calculators and other stationery are permissible.)
- Make sure you have the appropriate ID (photo ID, which is usually your student card or your passport).

and you lose concentration. If you start to lose concentration then it might be time for a short break, perhaps 10–15 minutes. This should be worked into your revision plan.

Other tips for improving concentration include switching to a different topic or mixing between topics you consider interesting or relatively boring. Also check that your environment is optimal, or maybe even take a short nap.

During periods of revision, you should also make sure you get enough sleep as lack of sleep is known to affect concentration and performance. To ensure a good night's rest ensure you keep and stick to a regular bed time, that you 'switch off' before going to bed (do something totally different to keep your mind off studying, and preferably at least an hour before going to bed), and that you avoid any stimulants or sedatives that will affect your sleep (caffeine, stimulant drinks, alcohol). On the day before the exam make sure you get enough sleep and try to resist the temptation to cram in lots of information as you may wear yourself out and so not perform efficiently.

Pre-examination checklist

Before you even go to the exam make sure you have everything you need; a checklist you might find useful is given in Box 8.1. Ideally, this should not be done on the day of the exam itself.

In summary, you may never feel totally prepared for an exam no matter how much preparation time you have put in, so it is best to focus on what the question is asking you. Also remember that you do not have to give perfect answers. Exams are not designed to fail students and most people end up passing most of the time.

Sitting the exam and tackling papers effectively

Sitting in the examination room waiting to start the exam is typically the period of highest tension and anxiety. Therefore you need to focus your thoughts on what you are about to do, relax yourself by taking some deep breaths, and try not to be distracted by the students around you.

When the exam starts, take some time to settle down and make sure you read each question carefully, especially when there is a choice of question to be made. What sometimes

Box 8.2 Some general tips for answering multiple-choice questions

- Find out whether you must use a pen or pencil.
- Circle or underline important words/sentences in the question.
- Read all the answer choices before selecting one and cross out those you are certain are incorrect.
- Look for two answer choices that are opposites as one of these is likely to be the correct answer.
- Do not change your initial answer unless you are sure another answer choice is correct. More often than not, your first choice is the right one.
- Is there negative marking? Sometimes there's nothing to lose by guessing, but if there is negative marking for an incorrect answer then it's safest to leave the answer grid blank for that question.

helps is to underline the key words/sentences in a question. Watch out for words such as 'discuss', 'illustrate', 'show with examples', and 'justify', as these will require you to include more in-depth explanations in your answer. This is different to words such as 'list' or 'state', which usually require lists of information (as bullet points) or factual statements, respectively. Underlining key words also serves to keep you on track when answering the question. (We discuss the interpretation of essay questions in more detail in Chapter 5.)

Remember, a common fault is for a student to fail to actually answer the question because either they have not understood it, or they have ignored important pieces of information in the question. Thus, it is best not to have preconceived ideas about what an answer to a particular topic is; don't launch straight into writing, without actually looking at what has been asked for. Also, try not to just write down everything you know about a topic if it does not answer the question asked. This shows a lack of understanding and interpretation, and will not get you any extra marks.

If you get stuck on a question or your mind goes blank, take a deep breath and decide whether your time would be better spent on another question. Getting stuck on a question can be a big time waster, so it is best to move on and then come back to the problematic question once you have completed the others. Also, make sure you keep track of time. Ideally, you need to factor in some time to check over your answers, as this can sometimes save you some marks. On that note, avoid leaving the exam early, even if you have finished: if there's time to spare, use it to check your answers.

Boxes 8.2 and 8.3 provide specific tips for answering MCQs and essays in the exam, respectively.

 Box 8.3 Some general tips for dealing with long-answer/essay questions

- Read each exam question through at least twice.
- Underline key words/sentences.
- Decide on the order you will answer the questions. If there is a 'compulsory' question, start with that one.

- Write an essay plan and before writing the actual essay go through the plan and revise it if necessary. It is best to check your plan addresses what the question is asking before jumping in and writing down everything you know in an incoherent manner. Answer the question, not what you think the question is.

- Check your answers. Read through what you have written to ensure you are happy with it. Check for spelling mistakes and grammatical errors.

- Remember that it is the quality of the argument/answer that matters, not the quantity of information provided.

- Make sure you clearly cross through the essay plan; however, you should ensure it is still legible in case you have missed anything out of your main answer, as the marker may possibly be able to give some marks for what was in your plan.

Managing expectations and minimizing anxiety

Feeling stressed or becoming anxious before and during an exam is a common occurrence, and is entirely normal and natural, especially as you will be thinking about whether you have prepared enough, or if you will remember enough to pass the exam. Typical indicators for anxiety include:

- feelings of irritability;
- heart palpitations;
- muscle tension;
- headaches;
- nausea, dizziness;
- shallow breathing;
- excessive sweating;
- change in sleep or eating habits.
  (Source: NHS Choices, 2015.)

Worrying can stop you from concentrating—the opposite of what you need when trying to complete an exam. There are various steps that you can take to help reduce stress, the first of which is starting revision early and sticking to your revision plan. If you think you are getting anxious or stressed then the following tips may help:

- Allow yourself some time to deal with what you are feeling. Take a few deep breaths and try to relax some muscles.

- Think about the cause of anxiety and potential solutions. We have already talked about what to do if you get stuck on a question.

- Think to yourself that the anxiety is unnecessary (keep things in perspective) and needs to stop, and that you can handle the situation.

- Believe in yourself.
- Try some relaxation techniques or do some exercise.
- If the stress or anxiety is continuous, take steps to overcome the problem. For example, speak to your tutor, friends, or family. If it is affecting your general well-being seek some help from the university counselling services or your doctor.
- It is important to seek help from the exam invigilators if you feel you can't control your anxiety within the exam.

In conclusion, preparing for and sitting exams does not have to be an ordeal if enough thought, time, and effort are applied to the task at hand. Following some of the hints and tips described above may be able to help you achieve success in your exams, but it is important to find out what works best for you and then stick with it. Preparation is vital so do not leave things to the last minute!

 Real-practice example

The following is an example of planning how long to spend on an exam. Suppose the exam:

- is a 3-hour exam;
- has 30 MCQs (section A);
- has three short-answer questions (10 marks each; section B);
- and has a choice of two from three essays (20 marks each; section C).

So, for a 3-hour exam, which equates to 180 minutes:

- 18 minutes for each 10 marks;
- 54 minutes for section A
  - 30 questions, so < 2 minutes per question;
- 54 minutes for section B
  - three questions, so 18 minutes each;
- 72 minutes for section C
  - two questions, so 36 minutes each.

In practical terms, don't forget that the times indicated should also incorporate a few minutes for planning and checking your answers (mainly sections B and C).

 Key points

- To pass an exam, you need to have a good knowledge and understanding of the material you are being examined on.
- Make yourself familiar with the types of questions you are likely to encounter. Look at past or sample exam papers for the format and question types used.

- Prepare a revision timetable. Be realistic about the amount of time you have to revise. Start early and ensure you factor in time for breaks.

- Ensure you create the most productive environment for revision.

- Try a range of study techniques to find what works for you. Visual aids and study groups can be effective methods if used correctly.

- Make sure you know when the exams are and go over your pre-exam checklist.

- Try and relax yourself before starting to answer the paper. Take some time to read through the paper, underline key words/sentences, and ensure you monitor your progress during the exam. Allow time for double-checking your answers.

- After the exam, it's best to avoid any sort of post-mortem analysis. Take a break and get mentally prepared for the next exam.

 Further reading and references

Azzopardi LM. MCQs in Pharmacy Practice. 2nd rev. ed. London: Pharmaceutical Press; 2009.

Bukhari N, Elsaid, N. Registration Exam Questions III (Tomorrow's Pharmacist). 1st ed. London: Pharmaceutical Press; 2014.

Cottrell S. The Study Skills Handbook. 3rd ed. Basingstoke: Palgrave MacMillan; 2008.

Evans BW, Kravitz L, Walker N, Lefteri K. Pharmacy OSCEs: A Revision Guide Paperback. 1st ed. London: Pharmaceutical Press; 2013.

Inglott AS, Azzopardi LM. MCQs in Clinical Pharmacy. 1st ed. London: Pharmaceutical Press; 2007.

NHS Choices (2015). *Stress, Anxiety and Depression* [online]. Available from: http://www.nhs.uk/conditions/stress-anxiety-depression/pages/understanding-panic.aspx [Accessed 20 October 2016].

Rowntree D. Learn How to Study: A Realistic Approach. 4th rev. ed. London: Sphere; 1998.

 Answers to the example questions

Example 1

1. Insulin is important in the regulation of blood glucose levels (True).

2. Aspirin has antiplatelet activity (True).

3. A cough suppressant is the best recommendation for treating a chesty cough (False).

Example 2

Answer is A: the professional qualifications of the prescriber.

Example 3

The best answer would be metformin because it is used as a first-line treatment and is recommended to be used in patients who are obese. Insulin does not fit the patient profile, gliclazide can cause weight gain so is not good for obese patients, acarbose is not recommended as first-line treatment, and sitagliptin could be used but only if the patient cannot tolerate metformin.

Example 4

Responses A, B, and E are true.
Responses C and D are false.

Example 5

Answer is E (3 only): have specific standard operating procedures in place.
You don't have to have an NHS contract to register the pharmacy and you can still stay open without a Responsible Pharmacist being present but are limited to the services that the pharmacy can provide.

Example 6

A 7-year-old boy who suffers from asthma has developed a high fever, as well as a runny nose. The boy has no known allergies and hasn't taken analgesics before.

Answer is E: paracetamol (paracetamol liquid is the recommended and safest option for a 7-year-old. All non-steroidal anti-inflammatory drugs (NSAIDs) should be used with caution in asthmatics, and an opioid analgesic would not be used to treat a fever).

A 50-year-old woman has chronic pain from bone cancer. She has completed her course of chemotherapy and is now under palliative care. She has allergies to morphine salts. She has been using tramadol at the maximum recommended dose, but this is no longer controlling her pain.

Answer is D—oxycodone tablets (patient needs a stronger analgesic than tramadol, which rules out NSAIDs and paracetamol. She is also allergic to morphine salts, which rules out morphine, and pethidine injection would not be used for this indication).

Example 7

Answer is E. Both statements are false—records should not be made in the CD register and an authorized witness is not legally required for destroying the drug, but it is preferable that one is present.

Statement 1	Statement 2
An entry needs to be made in the Controlled Drugs (CD) Register for patient-returned Schedule 2 controlled drugs	It is a legal requirement for patient-returned Schedule 2 controlled drugs to be destroyed in the presence of an authorized witness

Example 8

You are working in a pharmacy and assume the role of the responsible pharmacist. You decide to go out for lunch, leaving the pharmacy without a pharmacist. While away on lunch, a customer comes into the pharmacy to collect their dispensed prescription. Is your dispenser allowed to give out the prescription? Justify your answer.

Answer is 'no'. Justification is that handing over of dispensed medicines to a patient, patient representative, or delivery person needs to take place under the supervision (pharmacist to be able to advise and intervene, if necessary) of a pharmacist, and the supervising pharmacist will need to be physically present at the premises.

9

Working with others

 ## Overview

In this chapter we will discuss why working with others is particularly important for pharmacists, and how to do so most effectively. During the course of your study you will be given many opportunities to work with others, whether as part of a team during group work activities, or during placements. The skills required to work with others is pivotal to working in modern health care. Indeed, the Francis report that resulted from high-profile cases such as the failure in care at Mid Staffordshire NHS Trust made it clear that more effective and efficient integration of care is a major priority. Patients and service users have also expressed a strong desire for a more streamlined and unified approach to their health care. However, such a unified approach is particularly challenging to achieve in practice when you think about the different health care practitioners involved in the delivery of that care. One way that integrated care can be promoted is through inter-professional learning and finding effective ways to work with others.

So, what do we mean by 'working with others'? You can think about this in several ways—acting as a lead, or when coordinating or collaborating with others on work activities. It is not limited to just being a member of a team; it extends to being a leader or supervisor, which in a pharmacy setting would mean being a pre-registration tutor or pharmacy manager. Most jobs require you to work as part of a team, and if you can demonstrate with examples to a prospective employer how you have successfully worked with others, this will benefit your application.

 ## Learning outcomes

You should be able to demonstrate knowledge and understanding of the following after working through this chapter:

- the professionalism, communication, and interpersonal skills needed when working with others;
- working in teams and team roles;
- the importance of inter-professional education within the health care setting;
- hints and tips regarding managing, working, and solving problems within a team;
- different group-work activities.

Professionalism and appropriate behaviour

As a pharmacist you will be working closely with patients, often on a one-to-one basis. They will be looking to you for support and advice. As such, acting in a professional manner and maintaining clear professional boundaries is essential. The Royal Pharmaceutical Society provides guidance on professionalism and professional boundaries, which would be useful for you to read (see also Chapter 1).

Professionalism and appropriate behaviour also extends to working as part of a team. You will need to know who all the different people involved in the care of a patient are, and how they interact and collaborate with each other while working as a team. Basic politeness, courtesy and respect are fundamental to professionalism.

Interpersonal skills and communication

Interpersonal skills are the life skills we use every day to interact with other people, and include elements of communication, listening, problem solving, negotiating and decision-making. Communication, both orally and in writing, is a key skill when working with others. Aligned to this is the ability to listen and respond appropriately to what others say. Qualities such as empathy, reliability, confidence, and being able to influence others are important attributes (see also Chapter 1). People who have worked on developing strong interpersonal skills are usually more successful in both their professional and personal lives.

Being able to communicate effectively enables you to take part in discussions and present complex information; cooperate with others in personal, learning, and working situations; respond appropriately to the views and feelings of others; and offer support and encouragement, and help resolve conflict. In most cases when working with others, oral communication is more prominent. However, in some cases being able to communicate effectively in writing is just as important—for example, when producing minutes of a meeting, setting terms and conditions, writing standard operating procedures, and so on. We will go over some of these skills throughout the subsequent sections. However, these skills are not something you can learn from a book, but require continual practice, reflection, and feedback, and may take a long time to master.

The following points are good starting places for developing effective communication:

1. Think about the individual or group with whom you are communicating; what is their level of understanding likely to be? Are you using appropriate terminology? For example, the language in which you describe the action of a new drug to a patient for whom English is not their first language is likely to be very different to the description you give to a medical consultant or a nurse.

2. Demonstrate clearly that you are listening—e.g. by nodding your head or making small verbal comments such as 'yes' or 'okay'. Don't forget to think about body language or facial expressions, too. Smiling is a great way to influence the atmosphere within the team, or during consultations with patients.

3. Don't interrupt anyone while they are speaking. Allow them to get their point across before you make yours.

4. Think about what the person said and what they really mean. What do they really want you to hear or to know?

5. Don't be afraid to ask questions to check you have heard and understood correctly.

6. Leave silences. These enable other people to enter the conversation or give people the time to think about what was said.

7. Acknowledge all that has just been said and make sure discussion of that point has been concluded before changing the subject.
8. Give praise and thanks where possible.

Common group-based learning strategies

There will be a variety of situations in which you will be required to work in groups or teams, some of which have already been alluded to elsewhere in this book. The most common active learning teaching formats that you will likely encounter within pharmacy include problem-based learning (PBL), case-based learning (CBL), and team-based learning (TBL).

PBL is a form of education that is increasingly being used in health care professional courses. In its simplest form, PBL uses problems (patient-oriented problems in the case of health care) as a context for students to gain knowledge about a subject area/topic. It is a method of learning that combines aspects of collaborative and self-directed learning, and is facilitated by a tutor.

In PBL, students are typically presented with a case or scenario and they work in small groups to identify any aspects they do not understand. These are considered the students' own learning objectives. The students then carry out independent, self-directed research to find explanations to their learning objectives and then return to their groups to discuss their acquired information and knowledge. This process can happen several times to secure more information and to keep probing more deeply into the problem. Students then present their work (report or oral presentation), with feedback provided by their peers or tutor on the whole process. As such, PBL is clearly defined and follows a series of steps. It is important to note that the work is more student-led and the role of the tutor is to only facilitate the session—that is, to help guide students rather than impart knowledge or tell the students what to do.

This type of teaching method allows you to learn by working with problems. It aims to help you apply and integrate your existing knowledge and to identify and fill gaps in your knowledge. PBL also encourages you to develop essential skills in problem solving, self-directed learning, and teamwork. The outcome of this kind of teaching is the development of clinical-reasoning skills and an ability to apply deductive reasoning to a problem. It also challenges you with situations that you may encounter in your professional career.

In the case of pharmacy, the self-directed learning, small group work, and development of critical thinking can help you prepare for continuing professional development (CPD), which is a requirement for all pharmacists. CPD is a cyclical process of reflection on practice, planning, action, and evaluation (reflection on learning). It may include anything that a pharmacist learns which makes them better able to do their job.

CBL has some similarities to PBL but differs in a number of ways. It is a particular method of teaching that is based on the principles of PBL but places more emphasis on putting student learning into practice using realistic scenarios. Typically, clinical cases are used within sessions; these resemble—or are directly drawn from—real-world examples. The latter use of practical examples, as opposed to theoretical situations, helps students understand what they need to do and know, for their clinical practice.

CBL requires prior knowledge of content by the student, with learning objectives that are more clearly defined and consistent, and students are expected to review and apply their existing knowledge. Similarly to PBL, CBL promotes discussion, helps students apply analytic skills, and allows opportunities to reflect on their relevant experiences, and draw conclusions they can relate to new situations. The tutor in CBL has a more involved role than in PBL and will direct what the students should learn about the case—for example, by providing all the information in a previous lecture or by eliciting learning objectives through discussion.

TBL is being increasingly used in various higher education settings and involves a specific sequence of individual work, group work, and immediate feedback to create an environment in which students increasingly hold each other accountable for coming to class prepared (e.g. by attending a lecture or reading some journals) and for contributing to the discussion. Typically, during the first TBL session students take an individual readiness assurance/ assessment test (RAT) covering the preparatory work given. After this individual test, students retake the same test as a team, and immediately get feedback on how they scored on both the individual and team test. The individual tests hold students accountable for learning the material before the session and the team tests provide an opportunity for students to learn from one another while working together on the test.

The bulk of the session time is used to practise applying content, rather than acquiring it, in a series of team exercises. For example, each team is assigned a complex case representing a real-world problem, which requires them to use the materials they learnt as preparatory work. Each team has to work together then reveal their answer simultaneously, so feedback is immediate.

Common to all the active learning group formats highlighted is the need to work in teams, so the following sections of the chapter will show you how to get the best out of group/team-based activities.

Relationships within groups

As a student you will be typically working on a project or an assignment with others, either in pairs or in a group. Examples may include laboratory practicals, the development of posters, oral presentations, problem- or team- or case-based learning, and the development of pharmaceutical care plans. In all of these cases, you will be learning about the task or project that you have been set while simultaneously learning about how to work with your peers. The methods you use to communicate and work together will also depend upon the work you are assigned to do.

Working with others requires an ability to plan, organize, carry out, and reflect on your work. Knowing your strengths and weaknesses can influence how you work within a group and what role you are likely to play. Each member of a group influences how that group operates, even if only by remaining silent. The overall success of the group depends largely on whether everyone is prepared to take some responsibility for how the group operates and whether everyone feels free to contribute fully. This can be quite challenging to achieve and more often than not there is some imbalance in work ethic and contributions.

Team roles

The subject of team roles has been studied extensively over the last couple of decades. Arguably, the most popular studies are those carried out by Meredith Belbin, who developed the notion of clusters of behaviour that relate to an individual's natural tendencies in the way they interrelate with others. Belbin's self-scoring Self Perception Inventory was developed to help bring about improvements in individual and team performance. It asks questions such as how you believe you can make positive contributions to a team, explores why you may find it difficult to work in a team, your approach to working in a team, and how you go about resolving any issues. The model then classifies you according to the traits shown in Table 9.1. You may come across this model on your course when talking about teamwork or during interprofessional education (IPE). Additionally, some employers use this during team-building exercises. However, it should be noted that this test, along with the Myers–Briggs Type Indicator® mentioned below, is not scientifically validated and as such should not be taken as a serious indication of your personality type. For a fun look at your team role contribution you can undertake a free online test based on Belbin's model at https://www.123test.com/team-roles-test/.

As mentioned above, another exercise that some people use to examine psychological (personality) types when looking at team dynamics is called the Myers–Briggs Type Indicator® (MBTI®). The theory is that variation in behaviour to a situation is due to basic differences in the ways individuals prefer to use their perception and judgement. MBTI uses your

Table 9.1 Belbin's self-perception team roles and descriptions

Team role contribution	Descriptions
Plant	Creative, imaginative, unorthodox. Solves difficult problems. However, too pre occupied with own thoughts to communicate effectively.
Resource investigator	Extrovert, enthusiastic, communicative. Explores opportunities. Develops contacts. However, over-optimistic, and can lose interest once initial enthusiasm has passed.
Co ordinator	Mature, confident. Clarifies goals and brings other people together to promote team discussions. However, can be seen as manipulative and offloads personal work.
Shaper	Challenging, dynamic, thrives on pressure. Has the drive and courage to overcome obstacles. However, prone to provocation and liable to offend others.
Monitor evaluator	Serious minded, strategic, and discerning. Sees all options. Judges accurately. However, can lack drive and ability to inspire others.
Team worker	Co operative, mild, perceptive, and diplomatic. Listens, builds, averts friction. However, indecisive in crunch situations.
Implementer	Disciplined, reliable, conservative in habits. A capacity for taking practical steps and actions. However, somewhat inflexible and slow to respond to new possibilities.
Completer finisher	Painstaking, conscientious, anxious. Searches out errors and omissions. Delivers on time. However, inclined to worry unduly and reluctant to let others into own job.
Specialist	Single-mind, self-starting, dedicated. Provides knowledge and skills in rare supply. However, contributes only on a limited front. Dwells on specialized personal interests.

Source: http://www.belbin.com.

preferences to identify and describe 16 different personality types. The preferences are themselves derived from asking the following questions.

- Do you prefer to focus on the outer world (*Extraversion—E*) or on your own inner world (*Introversion—I*)?
- Do you prefer to focus on the basic information you take in (*Sensing—S*) or do you prefer to interpret and add meaning (*Intuition—I*)?
- When making decisions, do you prefer to first look at logic and consistency (*Thinking—T*) or first look at the people and special circumstances (*Feeling—F*)?
- In dealing with the outside world, do you prefer to get things decided (*Judging—J*) or do you prefer to stay open to new information and options (*Perceiving—P*)?

When you decide on your preference, you have your own personality type, which can be expressed as a code with four letters. For example:

ISTJ: *Quiet, serious, earn success by thoroughness and dependability. Practical, matter-of-fact, realistic, and responsible. Decide logically what should be done and work toward it steadily, regardless of distractions. Take pleasure in making everything orderly and organised—their work, their home, their life. Value traditions and loyalty.*

INTJ: *Have original minds and great drive for implementing their ideas and achieving their goals. Quickly see patterns in external events and develop long-range explanatory perspectives. When committed, organise a job and carry it through. Sceptical and independent, have high standards of competence and performance—for themselves and others.*

ESTP: *Flexible and tolerant, they take a pragmatic approach focused on immediate results. Theories and conceptual explanations bore them—they want to act energetically to solve the problem. Focus on the here-and-now, spontaneous, enjoy each moment that they can be active with others. Enjoy material comforts and style. Learn best through doing.*

ENTP: *Quick, ingenious, stimulating, alert, and outspoken. Resourceful in solving new and challenging problems. Adept at generating conceptual possibilities and then analysing them strategically. Good at reading other people. Bored by routine, will seldom do the same thing the same way, apt to turn to one new interest after another.*

(Source: The Myers & Briggs Foundation.)

MBTI can be used to gather and help analyse information about teams or groups of people. None of the personality types are considered better than others and part of the purpose of using the instrument is understanding that people have different preferences, views, and interests; behave differently; and are motivated by different things. Knowing about personality types is said to help you to understand, value, and appreciate differences between people, an important attribute to have when working within, or leading, a team or group activity. See the further reading section if you are interested in learning more about MBTI and finding out your own personality type.

As a member of a team it is very important to realize that the actions of every individual will impact on the team as a whole. The way you work affects everyone else and it is worth considering what your expectations are, and what teamwork traits you would want or not want. For example, think about how you would feel if you worked with someone who was disorganized, or late all the time, or did not do their task in the designated time. Would you be happy with this? If not, then don't act in this way yourself.

Tolerance of others in your team is quite important and not everyone will be seen as a team player. You need to be mindful of reasons why someone may not be seen to be a team player, for example they lack confidence, or see themselves as different owing to gender, race, age, language, or culture. This might even be you, and these types of issues and behaviours affect how you and others work and your relationships with your team members.

Effective group work

When working in a group, it is generally best to establish some ground rules at the outset. This is best done by ensuring that the group brainstorms, discusses, and agrees a set of rules. Once the ground rules are established each member of the group should receive a copy, which can be seen as a contract that everyone has to abide to. It should be made clear, and agreed, as to what the consequences of the ground rules being broken are.

Points to think about when setting ground rules are:

- Who will act as team leader and what will their responsibilities be? For example, will they be required to coordinate and lead the meetings? Will they send reminders about deadlines? Do they make the final decisions? This is sometimes best done on a rotational basis if the group is to meet on several occasions.

- If there are multiple meetings, everyone should agree to attend all meetings, and provide reasons for any absences.

- What are the roles and responsibilities of everyone else?

- Everyone should agree to contribute to the work and get an equal share of time when discussing matters. One way of doing this is to allow different people to go first or last each time.

It is often noticeable that some members of a group are more vocal or opinionated than others, are more active or less active than others, or are academically weaker or stronger than others. However, a good team has members with different strengths who can make different contributions. Recognizing these differences is important at an early stage. All team members should be included in discussions: everybody counts. Implicit in this is that individual interests should not come first; it is the desired outcome for the team that counts.

Self-reflection (thinking about your own needs, what you have gained, what you need to know or do) will enable you to get the best out of teamwork by guiding your expectations for what you want to achieve as part of a team, and how best you could contribute to the benefit of all your team members. It is part of CPD, which has already been mentioned elsewhere, and also plays an important role when working with others. Identifying ways of further improving your skills in this area will make working with others more enjoyable and productive.

Unfortunately, and inevitably, there will be some disagreements and how you handle these will be discussed later on.

At this stage, it is worth mentioning the submission of group work for assessment. When working together on a piece of assessed coursework as part of the group exercise, there is always the danger of ending up with the same piece of work among your team members, such that you may be accused of colluding (i.e. handing in work that closely resembles a friend's or is in greater part taken from a friend's work can constitute collusion) or plagiarizing (taking someone else's work or ideas and passing them off as one's own). Most courses now use a tool such as Turnitin to look for signs of plagiarism. It provides a similarity index between your work, other students' work within the university, and external sources (via the Internet), and so it is easier to detect signs of collusion and plagiarism. (We consider how to avoid collusion and plagiarism in Chapter 5.)

Unfortunately, working in groups, where information is sometimes gathered independently then shared, can increase the chance that problems are picked up. Just be extra vigilant and ensure your assessed work is as individual as possible.

Working with your 'boss'

When it comes to placements and projects (e.g. your research project), you will be managed by a tutor or a supervisor. Under these circumstances how you deal with your 'boss' is not unlike the team working dynamic we have already talked about above: it is important to employ strong communication skills and understand what is important to them. 'Managing upwards' is a routine term used in the corporate world to describe how an individual influences the behaviour of their 'boss' in a way that ensures a positive experience for the individual concerned.

Rather than using 'boss' we will now use the term 'tutor' to better fit the situations you will encounter during your studies. There are various things you may need to consider to ensure you engage effectively with your tutor.

- Understand your tutors' objectives. If you are on a placement, what do they want from you and how does this fit with the company's objectives? If it's your project supervisor, what do they want from the project (data for a publication, preliminary data)?

- Keep your tutor informed of your day-to-day activities, especially if any issues arise. This is particularly important if you are working on a ward or in a laboratory.

- Don't expect your tutor to give detailed guidance on absolutely everything. For example, for your research project the expectation would be for you to come up with options with your tutor and to make decisions under your tutor's guidance.

- Be honest and realistic about when you can complete a particular task. Failing to meet deadlines is not a good work ethic.

- Try not to argue with your tutor or confront them about a problem. As we will mention later, communicate your issues or concerns in a constructive, collaborative way.

- If you receive criticism from your tutor try to see this as a way to do better, not as a personal attack. React logically and not emotionally or defensively. Taking some time to think and reflect is always a good idea before responding to criticism.

- It may also be a good idea to find out about what they like or dislike regarding work practices. Does your tutor expect you to be punctual to meetings or at work? Do they expect you to write minutes for every meeting? Is poor grammar and spelling tolerated by them? Attention to such matters is a key aspect of professionalism and will help maintain a good working relationship.

We consider how to deal with your tutor if they are difficult to handle in the section 'Managing conflict and resolving differences'. If you find your tutor's behaviour is something that you can't manage then you may need to seek advice from your personal tutor, senior tutor, or head of department.

Learning in groups and inter-professional working

Numerous publicized reports over the last 10 years have highlighted breakdowns in health and social care services to individuals or groups of patients and service users. We have already mentioned the Mid Staffordshire NHS Foundation Trust case, which concluded that patients were routinely neglected and that the Trust was preoccupied with cost cutting, targets, and processes rather than its fundamental responsibility to provide safe patient care. Several health care professionals were found wanting in the level of care provided. What these reports have identified is a need for better collaborative, multi professional working in order to provide the best patient care. This starts at the level of education and training for health care professionals.

Various studies have looked at learning with other professionals, and have employed different terminology to describe it—for example, 'common learning', 'shared learning', 'multi-professional learning', and 'inter-professional education/learning (IPE/L)'. The meaning of these terms varies, but for true multi professional engagement and learning to occur, IPE is the preferred term. IPE is when two or more professionals learn with, from, and about each other. This should not be confused with multi professional learning, which is when two or more professions learn the same content alongside each other (also called 'shared learning').

It is generally well recognized (although evidence is lacking) that IPE is an integral part of developing efficient and collaborative working practices in a multidisciplinary team setting, such as that experienced in health care. Within the health care setting, the professionals involved in patient care can include medical doctors, dentists, physiotherapists, nurses, pharmacists, and others. For most of the professions involved, including pharmacy, their respective professional body requires some form of IPE to exist within their teaching and learning curriculum with a view to help improve patient care. Consequently, there is a strong desire to undertake IPE within professional courses.

From a pharmacy perspective, there are many opportunities for hospital pharmacists to interact inter-professionally as they participate on ward rounds and are involved in discussions around patient care. Community pharmacists face a different picture as they are more likely to work in isolation. However, with current changes in the National Health Service and the way in which community pharmacies are actively being asked to be involved in patient-care pathways, there is a strong need to encourage better inter-professional interaction to provide the best care for patients.

So what benefits can IPE provide? IPE helps to manage relationships between the growing numbers of professions, and, ultimately, it can improve patient safety by improving communication and collaboration between professions. It has been noted that pharmacy students have found learning with other professions to be powerful experiences, which affect their attitudes and values and also enhance their knowledge and skills for the development of team and collaborative working (Anderson and Lennox, 2005). Therefore, as you learn with, from, and about other professions, barriers (such as prejudices and stereotypes) come down and mutual trust and respect develop, which should then lead to better quality of care for patients. Currently, there are positive moves to getting more pharmacists within general practitioner practices, and what seems to come across is that to work more effectively we need to understand and know about the needs of other professions and how we can interact best with them.

It may be that you have already had some experience of IPE within your course. Unfortunately, no uniform, national model of IPE exists for pharmacy students, and so content and delivery varies from one university to another. Some of the professions included in IPE activities are pharmacy, medicine, physiotherapy, nursing, dentistry, dieticians, chiropody, optometry, occupational therapy, nutrition, midwifery, and social work. A range of activities are undertaken, with some of the common ones listed below.

- Ice-breaking sessions within multidisciplinary professional teams (e.g. comparing and contrasting professional roles and responsibilities).

- Participating in team-based assignments (case- or problem-based learning, role plays), with opportunities to reflect on working relationships and experiences.

- Going on placements within the community or hospital settings. During the placement students either observe inter-professional working or partake in tasks that involve the development and application of inter-professional relationships with students from other professions (e.g. medicine).

- IPE conference days where patients, carers, and service users are able to tell students their story.

Whatever format is used to deliver IPE, the true value of it is to learn from and about others. If you are asked to be involved in any IPE activities, including going on a placement, take this opportunity to learn about others and also to teach others about your profession. The fewer barriers that exist to working with others, the better for everyone.

Managing conflict and resolving differences

Within the workplace setting, you will become a valuable member of the team if you actively seek to cooperate with all of your colleagues and work productively. However, as mentioned previously, there may be circumstances in which conflicts arise. These may arise from someone not being punctual, not attending meetings, not contributing to discussions or performing their allocated task, or even bullying and harassment. Bullying involves behaviour that can involve an imbalance of power and lead to either mental or physical damage to the person affected. Harassment or discrimination (mentioned briefly in Chapter 10) may be seen in different ways and usually involves issues of race, gender, age, or disability. Examples

Table 9.2 Different ways to deal with conflict and the merits and pitfalls for each

Action	Possible consequences
Deny or suppress the conflict	Only works if the real issue is adequately dealt with. If not, then there is the risk you will become resentful. Speaking up about issues that bother you in a diplomatic and respectful way will allow you to disagree without creating further bad blood
Accommodate, and yield to the other person	This can come out of the need to avoid conflict, or it can be due to the person's belief that their rights, feelings, or desires are not as important as those of others. Accommodating others' needs over yours all of the time is not workable in the long run
Feed the conflict	If you go out to win and show concern only for what you want then nobody really wins. Unless each person's concerns have been heard and their basic needs met in the solution to the conflict you cannot move forward to resolve the conflict
Compromise	Compromising is a general step in the right direction. However, compromise involves identifying something that both sides must give up, and so it is still not the ideal solution
Work with the other person to solve the problem mutually	This should be done in a way that recognizes and respects what each person wants. Learning to work with the other person means that you will always be aiming to achieve the best outcome in any conflict

of bullying or harassment include humiliating someone, heavy criticism, verbal or physical threats, inappropriate jokes, innuendo, and ignoring or freezing someone out.

Whatever the reasons, dealing with conflict can be a difficult process and the readiness with which you can do so can depend on your own background and personality. You may already have experiences of situations where a conflict arose. Can you remember what happened or how you dealt with it? Such reflection is important because thinking about how you respond to conflict tells you something about your style of dealing with negative situations. For example, do you avoid conflict? Do you get involved and try and keep the peace? Do you feed the conflict? Do you compromise? Table 9.2 shows different ways people deal with conflict.

A note of caution is that any conflict should not arise as a result of discrimination. The Equality Act 2010 applies to any workplace setting and looks at discrimination based on protected characteristics such as age, race, gender, pregnancy, religion or belief, sexual orientation, and disability. It would be a criminal offence if this law was broken. From a learning perspective (during your studies), discrimination would be grounds for suspension, or even removal from the course.

So what points should you consider to be able to resolve a conflict?

- Make sure you are clearly understood. Repeat the key points that you want people to think about.
- Everyone concerned should always be direct and open about their concerns.
- If the same problems are recurring on a regular basis, involve the rest of the group.
- Seek a solution to eliminate problems before they begin.
- Solve problems when they arise. This can be done by being objective: focus on the actual issues, rather than who did what, listen to what each person has to say, then brainstorm

to find the appropriate way to work together. Don't let a small problem grow into a bigger one.

- If you are not able to resolve a conflict then don't complain or moan about it to the rest of your group or friends. In the classroom setting it is best you speak to your class tutor and ask them to intervene. Within the work setting, this may be your line manager or supervisor.

In summary, working with others can be a challenging yet rewarding experience. You will come across this during your studies (group work, placements) and in your professional life. Where possible, through reflection, you will need to develop and improve your communication, interpersonal, and negotiation skills in order to not only contribute to an effective work environment, but also develop others, break stereotypes, and encourage seamless working practices. In the health care setting this will result in the best patient care, and during your studies, in a rewarding, and hopefully fun, learning experience.

 Key points

- There are many instances in your time at university, and especially in the work setting, when you will be required to work in a group or team and so you need to be able to make the most out of these learning environments.
- The most common group work activities include PBL, CBL, and TBL.
- Working in a group/team requires you to develop and apply a range of interpersonal skills. Reflecting on your own skill set will help you better prepare for group/team work.
- You should be aware of different personality types, including your own, when dealing with and working with others.
- Inter-professional education is key for future health care practice. Learning with, from, and about other health care professionals will mean better outcomes for patients.
- When working in a group make sure you set ground rules. This will help minimize any potential conflict among team members and ensure effective team working.
- When managing a conflict keep a level head and allow everyone involved to voice their concerns.

Examples of group-work activity settings

The following are examples of the types of classroom activities you may experience in your course. You could even use some of these yourself for practising role plays, brainstorming ideas, or for revision.

Think–pair–share/write–pair–share

This activity asks you to think individually about a particular question or scenario. After a few minutes, you pair up by either turning to your partner, or by forming small groups. You then discuss and compare your ideas. The responses are then shared within larger groups or with the entire class. The purpose behind this activity is to generate ideas, giving you a chance to validate your ideas with a small group before mentioning it to the whole class, which, in turn, can increase your confidence in your answers.

Fishbowl

This method involves one group/individual debating, advising, or talking about an issue with another group/individual, with a third person observing the whole process. Role plays fit this model where one person may be the pharmacist, one the patient, the other the observer. After the activity there is a debriefing with the observer providing feedback on how the process went. The process is typically repeated to allow each person to take on a different role.

Learning teams

Learning teams see you divided into groups at the beginning of the term. You then remain in these groups over the term or whole academic year. Any group work activity (e.g. as in case- or problem-based learning) is assigned to these pre-determined groups. This is usually a good way for you to get to know your team mates better, particularly if done in an inter-professional setting.

Circle of voices

This involves you and your fellow students taking turns to speak. You form circles of four or five and are given a topic, which you are allowed a few minutes to think about. Then the discussion starts, with each student having up to a few minutes of uninterrupted time to speak. After everyone has spoken once, the group has a general discussion, with the idea being that you should only build on what someone else has said, not on your own ideas. This type of activity helps you generate ideas and develop listening skills.

Snowball groups/pyramids

This method involves you first working alone, then in pairs, then in fours, and so on. As such, you come together with other students to discuss your ideas with the entire class. During each successive grouping it is usual to build upon an idea or be provided with increasingly complex tasks. The idea behind this type of activity is to generate well-examined ideas and develop your decision-making skills.

Jigsaw

This method introduces the concept of you becoming an 'expert' on one aspect of a topic. The group is provided with a topic, which is divided into a few parts or 'puzzle pieces'. Subgroups are then assigned a different piece of the puzzle in which they then go on to develop expertise. Once students have become experts they are moved around to form new groups. The students then take turns sharing their expertise with the new group members, until the puzzle is effectively solved. Sometimes this exercise may be performed over a few days or weeks, with the option of students doing research and developing the expertise outside of the classroom. This method is often very effective as it aids in-depth learning and gives you the opportunity to teach other students (learning from and about each other).

 ## References and further reading

Anderson E, Lennox A. The Leicester Model of Interprofessional Education: developing, delivering and learning from student voices for 10 years. J Interprof Care. 2009;23(6):557–573.

BELBIN®. *Belbin team roles* [online]. Available from: http://www.belbin.com [Accessed 8 April 2015].

Briggs Myers I. An Introduction to Type. A Guide to Understanding Your Results on the Myers Briggs Type Indicator. 6th ed. Oxford: Oxford Psychologists Press; 2000.

Burgess H. *Group projects: a conflict resolution guide for students. Beyond intractability* [online]. Available from: http://www.beyondintractability.org/educationtraining/group-projects [Accessed 24 October 2016].

Centre for Advancement of Interprofessional Education (CAIPE): http://caipe.org.uk

Harris TE, Sherblom JC. Small Group and Team Communication. 5th ed. London: Pearson; 2010.

Levin P. Successful Teamwork! For Undergraduates and Taught Postgraduates Working on Group Projects (Student-Friendly Guides Series). London: Open University Press; 2004.

Levine D, Wren M. *Working Together: Interactive Interprofessional Learning in the Classroom. MedEdPORTAL Publications* [online]. Available from: https://www.mededportal.org/publication/9329 [Accessed 24 October 2016].

The Myers & Briggs Foundation. *MBTI® Basics* [online]. Available from: http://www.myersbriggs.org/my-mbti-personality-type/mbti-basics [Accessed 28 July 2015].

Rawlinson, J. Creative Thinking and Brainstorming. Farnham: Gower Publishing Ltd; 1986.

Reeves S, Perrier L, Goldman J, Freeth D, Zwarenstein M. Interprofessional education: effects on professional practice and healthcare outcomes (update). Cochrane Database Syst Rev. 2013;3:CD002213.

Quine L. Workplace bullying in NHS community trust: staff questionnaire survey, *BMJ*. 1999;318(7178):228–232.

Woods J. 10 Minute Guide to Teams and Teamwork. Hungry Minds. New York: Macmillan Spectrum/Alpha Books; 1997.

10 Undertaking practice placements and reflection on practice

 Overview

An important part of your learning relates to the practical application of pharmacy knowledge in workplace settings. A UK-based course will provide you with the opportunity to attend pharmacy practice placements. As such, it is important for you to know how to best engage with such opportunities to maximize your learning.

A placement is the temporary posting of someone into a workplace to enable them to gain work experience. While some universities require students to complete an assessment element as part of a formal process, ideally you should also reflect on the impact of the placement on your wider personal and professional development.

In addition to the placements offered by your university, many workplaces offer short undergraduate pharmacy training posts during university closure periods, mainly during the summer months. A very strong argument can be made that a diligent student would seek this type of employment to help boost their personal portfolio, experience of pharmacy practice, and therefore future career prospects.

This chapter is about learning in practice settings and consolidating your learning. However, it also reflects the fact that you need to understand a number of formalities, including the need to respect confidentiality, to observe data protection rules, and to undergo criminal record disclosures, to work effectively within the pharmacy practice work setting.

As such, the chapter will discuss the sourcing of summer and other training posts; Disclosure and Barring Service checks, occupational health checks, health and safety; confidentiality, data protection, discrimination; engaging with practice placements; learning from practice placements and training posts; and reflecting on experiences.

 Learning outcomes

You should be able to demonstrate knowledge and understanding of the following after working through this chapter:

- how to source a pharmacy work experience or training post and meet the basic formal requirements for working in a pharmacy;
- how to engage actively with and learn from a practice workplace.

The importance of pharmacy placements

The majority of students who enrol onto a pharmacy degree course have the intention to work as a pharmacist upon qualifying. One of the steps towards qualification as a pharmacist is to complete formal pre-registration training either within the degree course or afterwards. At the time of writing this book, Health Education England was in the process of implementing a centralized system for the recruitment and allocation of formal pharmacy training posts in England. Regardless of the exact mechanism for managing the allocation of training places, it is worth noting that training posts are normally allocated on the basis of a formal application process, which includes a job interview. Recognized training posts are greatly sought after and oversubscribed, making them highly competitive. Even the less popular training posts are likely to be somewhat competitive. Therefore, as a student of pharmacy, you need to be able to make your individual job application stand out.

One of the ways to do this is to demonstrate prior experience within the pharmacy practice workplace setting. Pharmacists can work not only in hospitals or community pharmacies, but also increasingly in health centres, general practice settings, and clinical commissioning groups. Having demonstrable experience in a pharmacy setting, in whichever sector of practice, is important: it will enable you to show future employers that you have engaged with the workplace and can bring some experience and understanding of the real job of pharmacy to your post. Any job application would undoubtedly be strengthened by a record of your learning within such a placement.

There are many other reasons for pursuing pharmacy placements, too, including the opportunity to network with others, to increase your skills and knowledge in pharmacy, and to clarify in which sector you might want to pursue your career. Do not forget that working for someone also gives you a person who might be able to act as a referee for you in future job applications.

Sourcing summer and other training posts

It is outside of the scope of this book to provide large amounts of detail about job applications and job interviews—you would be advised to seek that level of guidance from your university's careers support service. Nonetheless, this section provides some important tips when seeking pharmacy practice posts. Whether you are looking for a short stint in a pharmacy during the holidays, a longer structured training post in the summer break, or, indeed, formal training preceding registration as a pharmacist, the first point to consider is where you might find information about any relevant training/job opportunities.

You can target employers speculatively by contacting them in the hope that they might be sufficiently impressed by your application to offer you a post. For example, if your aim is to seek a 2-week observation of practice in a community pharmacy on an unpaid basis, then you might well approach pharmacies local to where you live.

However, if you intend to apply for a structured training programme with one of the community pharmacy companies, then you will need to work more systematically. For example, you should find out which companies offer such training, the process of application, and deadlines for submitting them.

Similarly, you will need to familiarize yourself with the detail relating to the application process for gaining longer, recognized training posts. It is also a good idea to attend any careers fairs organized by your university so that you can meet employers and create your own contacts within the pharmacy industry.

Undoubtedly, formal job applications will require you to submit a curriculum vitae (CV) and covering letter and/or to complete a job application form. A CV, if you are not familiar with one, is a summary of your experience, skills, and education. It can be compiled using a text package such as Microsoft Word, although there are also electronic tools (CV builders) that can guide you through the process of constructing one.

Some people advocate keeping your CV to two pages, especially at undergraduate level, although the length and presentation of a CV can be dependent on the job role and the field of work. For example, most academics will keep a short CV, as well as a much larger CV—one of the authors' own full CV runs to around 30 pages! The standard information you should note on your CV is listed in Box 10.1.

If you are asked to complete a job application, you are likely to need to supply the standard information found on a CV. However, you might also be asked to write a personal statement

---

 Box 10.1   The standard information that should be noted on a CV

Personal details

Include your name, address, and contact details, including email address. Some people include age, marital status, and nationality, but this is not compulsory as they should not influence a decision about your suitability for the post. One important note is that your email address should sound professional and not create the wrong impression, for example 'foxylady@yahoo.co.uk' cannot possibly create the right impression! Some people add a link to their profile on a professional social media website such as LinkedIn, if they have one. Clearly, you would need to make sure that the webpage does not undermine your application in any way (e.g. your profile picture is suitable and projects a professional image).

Personal profile

Treat this as a short advertisement for you. Summarize your skills, your qualities, your background and achievements, and your career aims. You might want to steer clear of really generic words such as 'team player, conscientious, reliable', and so on—everyone uses them and they will not distinguish you from the next candidate. You might want to look at what the job specifically involves and then match your skills to the requirements; for example, good at handling conflict or excellent customer-care skills might be more useful skills to point out. Make sure that your career aims will chime with the job opportunity on offer, too.

Employment history and work experience

As an undergraduate you might have limited work experience to list here. You might want to consider including all relevant work experience, even if for a short duration or unpaid. Start with your most recent job and work backwards. Include here the name of your employer, the dates you worked for them, your job title, and your main duties and responsibilities. You might also want to provide more detail on what exactly you did, with examples of skills you gained or developed and your achievements. Some people advocate using positive verbs to describe your experience such as 'created, designed, established, supervised', and so on. Include the detail of any voluntary work, which can be highly regarded by some potential employers.

Once you start working after your degree, it becomes crucial not to leave unexplained gaps in your employment history, for example if you have taken time out to care for a relative or to travel, you must explain this along with what you learnt in that time. It is not wrong to take time out, but it is important to explain the reason.

Education and training

Use this section to list your most recent qualifications first. Then work back to the ones you got at school. Use a list or a table to include the name of the university, college or school you attended, the dates the qualifications were awarded, and your grades. If you have attended work-based courses then include these, too, if they are relevant.

Interests and achievements

If you have any interests or achievements that are relevant to the post then list them here. For example, you might judge that being a course representative for your pharmacy degree shows that you have been selected to a responsible position by others, demonstrating to your employer that you are capable of accepting responsibility. If you play a team sport, again that might equally demonstrate your ability to be an effective team member. Note that this section is not for listing general hobbies that have no relevance to the post. For example, swimming, dancing, or stamp collecting might not quite paint the picture you want to portray.

Additional information

If you have any other relevant information you can create a penultimate section and add the material here. For example, you might want to point out that you have a driving licence or that you speak a foreign language.

References

This section will list the names of people who can be contacted in order to provide an opinion about you and your suitability for the post advertised. At least one of your referees should be work related. If you have not yet gained work experience, then at least one should be an academic, for example your personal tutor. You should ideally make clear the relationship of your referee is to you clear—for example 'Dr Parastou Donyai, personal tutor'—together with their address, email address, and phone number. Do ask your referees if they agree to be named on your CV and do keep them informed of any job applications you are making so that they can anticipate any reference requests.

or answer shorter questions, to show how you meet the job description. Most posts formally advertised will include a job description that details the work itself, as well as a person specification, outlining the personal qualities sought. In reality, most employers want to see a similar set of skills and personal qualities: good communication, teamwork and interpersonal skills, self-management, organizational skills, and, of course, the potential to learn and perform the specific job.

When you write your personal statement or answer short questions about your suitability, make sure that you set out in a structured way how you meet the job description and person specification. For example, include your relevant skills and experience, ideally with specific examples so that your application stands out from the many other applications an employer is likely to receive (see Box 10.2). Your writing, of course, has to be clear and concise—there is nothing worse than job applications that ramble on or miss the point. A good proportion of job applications nowadays involve the completion of an online form. It is highly advisable that you print out and read a draft copy of the material you entered online to ensure that you

Box 10.2 Example answers to questions found on job application forms

Question: Why do you think you are suitable for this placement?

Suggested example answer:

I am a hard-working student who wants to gain structured training within a reputable pharmacy chain that offers exciting and innovative patient services. I have developed a number of skills during my degree course so far, including team working and problem solving; for example, I am currently working on a group project with six other students and we are all contributing towards designing a new pharmacy service. I also have some experience of working within the pharmacy sector through the structured placements that my university has organized, which has confirmed my passion for community pharmacy. I would make the absolute most of my summer training and would work to exceed all expectations if I were to be given the opportunity to join your company.

Question: Why do you want to work in hospital pharmacy?

Suggested example answer:

Hospital pharmacy is at the forefront of developing and delivering clinical pharmacy services, including cancer therapy, which I have a particular interest in. I have gained experience within both the community and hospital pharmacy sectors. I believe that a training post within a hospital pharmacy would align perfectly with my ambition to be a specialist consultant pharmacist in cancer chemotherapy in the future.

spot and correct any mistakes or spelling errors. Finally, if you can send in a covering letter, then do take advantage of this opportunity to specify to your future employer the skills you have and why you are the candidate they are looking for.

If your application is short-listed you might be invited to interview, or asked to attend an assessment centre for a structured test or to take a psychometric test, or a combination of all of these. The key to success is to find out as much detail as possible about the next steps and to prepare in advance. Box 10.3 lists a number of standard interview questions that you should know about and prepare answers for in advance of any interview.

Some employers use values-based questions as part of their recruitment process—for example during multiple mini-interviews. Multiple mini-interviews are, in essence, a series of stations through which candidates rotate, answering different questions at each. Values-based questions attempt to tease out candidates' personal values and behaviours to see if these align with that of the employer. Values-based questions can form a part of any type of recruitment process and not just multiple mini-interviews. The values of the National Health Service (NHS) constitution are shown in Figure 10.1. You can help demonstrate your

 Box 10.3 Standard interview questions and some tips to guide your preparation

Please describe yourself in one sentence/paragraph: *Make sure your answer is concise and interesting. For example, select one skill, characteristic, and success to highlight.*

Tell us why you applied for this job: *Select an example from your education and experience to demonstrate how you fit the company's ethos and the role advertised.*

What are your strengths (or, for example, what three words best describe you)? *Prepare by thinking of three key strengths (e.g. communicating with a range of people) and corresponding examples.*

What are your weaknesses (or, for example, how would someone you do not get on with describe you)? *Answer this question by picking a real example and showing how you have improved.*

If you were a medicine, what would you be (or, for example, if you were a car)? *Relate the medicine to an aspect of your personality, for example Gaviscon because you are good at soothing upsets!*

Provide an example of a time when you had to cope with a difficult situation. *Your example could relate to when, for example, you had to meet a short deadline or handle conflict.*

What has been your greatest achievement? *Ideally, show how you have used a set of key skills that contributed towards your success, for example organizing a student conference.*

If you had a bad experience with us during your training, how would you deal with it? *Do not become defensive or badmouth other organizations; instead, talk about following procedure.*

Where do you see yourself in 10 years (5 years/1 year)? *Show the relevance to the employers' goals and not just your own, for example becoming a consultant pharmacist or area manager.*

Tell us why we should hire you. *For example, how might you pass the registration exam or how might you work in a busy environment and help the employer meet its goals and targets?*

What questions would you like to ask us? *Do take this opportunity to ask sensible questions, for example what are my key targets in this role; what potential audits/projects can I contribute to?*

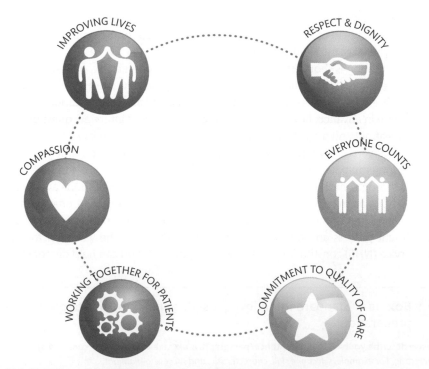

Figure 10.1 The values of the National Health Service (NHS) constitution.

Adapted from 'Values mapping tool' (http://www.nhsemployers.org/case-studies-and-resources/2014/04/values-mapping-tool).
© NHS Employers 2014.

Box 10.4 Examples of behaviours that demonstrate adherence to values in the National Health Service constitution

Give an example of how your behaviours demonstrate your commitment to the following values:

Working together for patients

Last year I undertook a placement in a small community pharmacy as part of my degree course. I was given a small dispensing task. Unfortunately, I made an error, which I picked up on and immediately told the pharmacist about. I then worked through my lunch hour to rectify my mistake so that it would not impact on the patient who was coming back that afternoon to collect their medication.

Respect and dignity

I realized after meeting with my personal tutor, and reflecting on my needs, that sometimes I interrupt a conversation to get my own point across, rather than listen to what the other person is trying to tell me. My tutor recommended that I read a book all about improving my listening skills. I read this and completed all the exercises. I now feel I really give my peers a chance to talk when we engage in discussions.

Everyone counts

There are people on my course of different ethnic backgrounds, ages, and abilities. At first, a group of us who were privately educated were avoiding the rest of the year group. When we were put into workshop groups according to surnames rather than friendship groups, I realized how much I could learn from people with a different perspective. Now I see that everyone has a point of view that is valid and should count.

Commitment to quality of care

We are given professional development folders to complete at university. This is seen as a burden by some of my peers. I have a completely different view of this. As far as I can see, I should commit to improving my knowledge and skills now and after my degree so that patient care is not compromised. I see the professional development folder as an opportunity to show my commitment to care quality.

Compassion

During the summer holidays I do some volunteering for a local charity shop. The charity helps people who have suffered a stroke. The shop also provides people who have suffered a stroke with an opportunity to work on a volunteer basis. When I am completing a shift with someone who has suffered a stroke, I make sure I am patient and understanding, for example where the person's speech has been affected.

Improving lives

My grandma lives near the university and we often talk about my experience on the course. She mentioned last Christmas that there are a lot of older people in the local community who would appreciate the opportunity to somehow get involved in helping students with their learning. I mentioned this to the head of pharmacy and now we have older people taking part in our workshops, to help students' communication skills.

suitability against the values listed in Figure 10.1 by giving examples of relevant behaviours. A number of such examples are provided in Box 10.4.

Sufficient preparation should give you the confidence to do yourself justice during the recruitment process.

Table 10.1 Examples of psychometric questions

Type of test	Example questions
Personality test	Likert scale: strongly agree—agree—neutral—disagree—strongly disagree
	Testing conscientiousness:
	I have almost never forgotten to show up for an appointment (ANSWER: a conscientious person would strongly agree)
	Testing extraversion:
	I like to be the centre of attention at a party (ANSWER: an extraverted person would strongly agree)
	Testing integrity:
	If someone is undercharged in a supermarket then they should tell the person at checkout (ANSWER: a person with high integrity would strongly agree)
	Testing leadership:
	The most successful people are those who have been inspired by a big idea or goal (ANSWER: a person with leadership skills would strongly agree)
Test of creativity	*Use of objects:*
	How many uses can you think of for a brick?
	(ANSWER: not just to build a wall/house, e.g. dinner table for mice!)
	Spotting associations:
	Find the link between 'wheel–electric–high'
	(ANSWER: 'chair', i.e. wheelchair, electric chair, highchair)
Intelligence test	*Verbal reasoning:*
	How many sports in LOOP? And what are they? (ANSWER 2; polo, pool)
	Numerical ability:
	What are the next two numbers in this sequence: 7, 11, 9, 14, 12, 18,...,... (ANSWER 16, 23)

It is outside of the scope of this chapter to cover psychometric tests in any detail, but if the recruitment process involves the completion of a psychometric test, then there are a couple of important points to note. Firstly, psychometric tests in the main aim either to explore your personality or your aptitude (see Table 10.1). Secondly, there is very little point in trying to 'cheat' a personality questionnaire. In addition, unless you have a lot of time to learn and prepare, it is very hard to 'revise' for an aptitude test. In any case, you would not want to give a distorted picture of yourself—it will not be much fun doing a job that you obtained on the basis of false answers! After all, the whole point of a psychometric test is to see if your character/attributes will fit the role and the organization.

Preparing for placements and training posts

There are a number of formalities to complete before starting most placements or training posts in the UK. Two important ones include the Disclosure and Barring Service (DBS) check (previously the Criminal Record Bureau check) and the occupational health check.

The DBS is, in effect, a criminal record check. Because working in a pharmacy practice setting will bring you in contact with patients, a number of employers, including the NHS, will request a DBS check before offering you a contract of employment. Note that there are three levels of check that can be carried out and that it can take up to 8 weeks to get a DBS check. The 'standard' DBS checks for spent and unspent convictions, cautions, reprimands, and final warnings. The 'enhanced' DBS is similar to the standard DBS but includes checks for additional information held by local police, which is reasonably considered relevant to the role. The 'enhanced with lists checks' is similar to the enhanced DBS but includes a check of the DBS barred lists—these contain the names of individuals who are unsuitable for working with children or adults and therefore cannot do certain types of work, including 'regulated activity'. The provision of health care by (or under the supervision of) a health care professional, including pharmacy professionals, is regulated activity. Therefore, the 'enhanced barred lists checks' is the DBS that will apply to you if you are asked to undertake a DBS check.

In addition, to undergo a DBS check you must be able to provide a range of original documents to prove your identity. Rather than listing these here, we would advise that you check the latest guidance online.

An occupational health check (also known as a work health assessment in the NHS) can also form a part of the pre-employment checks that you are asked to undertake after being offered a placement or training post. The purpose of this check is to identify if you have a health condition or disability that requires adjustments in the workplace (to allow you to undertake the role offered) or to identify if you have a health condition or disability that requires restriction of your role (e.g. avoiding certain activities in people with a blood-borne virus). Certainly the aim is not to discriminate against you. Note that some employers will want you to be fully up to date with your immunization status. This can result in you being asked to have any vaccines you had not previously received, administered before starting work.

To conclude this section, let us consider health and safety, the idea that your well-being should be protected while at work. There are many ways in which people's health and safety can be compromised at work. These include stress, exposure to chemicals or other hazardous substances, slips and trips, musculoskeletal disorders (e.g. through repetitive tasks such as computer use), noise, and so on.

Your employer or placement provider is responsible for your welfare while at work. For example, they should make you aware of fire exits and fire precautions on arrival, and provide you with guidance and training to complete relevant tasks. But you also have a duty to take care of yourself and the health and safety of other people who might be affected by your actions. To do this, you have to make sure that you listen carefully and follow any instructions that you have been given accurately, and take part responsibly in any training provided. You must use safety equipment (e.g. gloves) appropriately and also dispose of any hazardous material as instructed.

If during your placement or employment you have any concerns about health and safety then you must raise these with your placement organizer or employer. Certainly, you must report any accident or work-related illness as soon as you become aware of it. We would strongly advise you to read the factsheet 'Looking out for Work Hazards—Advice for Young People' referenced at the end of this chapter before embarking on a work placement or training post.

Confidentiality, data protection, and discrimination

Before you start your post or placement, it is helpful to think carefully about some other important expectations your employer/host will have in terms of your behaviour at work. One such expectation relates to confidentiality. If you spend any time in a pharmacy practice setting, however short, you are likely to come across various information sources that can identify a person as a patient or recipient of care, for example the patient's name, address, postcode, date of birth, media (e.g. photographs), NHS number, or other local identifiable code. Indeed, you might well be asked to collect such information from a patient, for example when offering a pharmacy service. It is important for you to respect a person's right to privacy and therefore treat any patient identifiable information in confidence. The confidentiality model outlines four requirements that have to be met to ensure that patients are provided with a confidential service. This model can be summarized as follows:

● PROTECT: look after the patient's information;

● INFORM: ensure that patients are aware of how their information is used;

● PROVIDE CHOICE: allow patients to decide whether their information can be disclosed or used in particular ways;

● IMPROVE: always look for better ways to protect, inform, and provide choice.
  (Adapted from Department of Health, 2003)

You should treat all information you receive during your placement or post in a confidential manner, be it relating to patients, the running of the business/premises, or any conversation that you may overhear. Needless to say, you should not engage in gossip, and you should be very careful about discussing a patient's case in a public space. Similarly, you should not take away with you (e.g. on a laptop or on paper) any notes that could be used to identify a patient. Instead, all files and equipment such as laptops should be locked away safely—or if you are collecting data for an audit, for example, you should fully anonymize any information you take off site—taking care to remove the patient's name, address, postcode, and any other detail or combination of details that might lead to identification.

There are many other ways in which you can keep patient information secure. Related to the idea of confidentiality is a concept known as data protection. The Data Protection Act specifies how personal information can be used by an organization. For example, information must be used fairly and lawfully, for a specifically stated purpose, not kept for longer than is necessary, be kept safe and secure, and so on. You should make sure that you read any lecture notes or guidance you have been given by your university about confidentiality and data protection before embarking on your pharmacy practice experience. During your placement or post, if you are in any doubt about the processing of patient data, then you should ask someone in authority for clarity.

A final behaviour to consider is discrimination. It is against the law to treat someone differently because of their age, sex, sexual orientation, transgender status, being married or in a civil partnership, being pregnant or having a child, disability, race (colour, nationality, ethnic or national origin), and religion (belief or lack of). These are known as 'protected characteristics'. People are protected from discrimination at work, in education, as a consumer, when using public services, when buying or renting property, and as a member or guest of a private club or association. People are also protected from discrimination if they are associated with someone who has a protected characteristic (e.g. a relative), or they have complained about discrimination or supported someone else's claim.

As a placement student or trainee you must therefore make sure that you do not discriminate against anybody. This can include direct discrimination—that is, treating someone with a protected characteristic less favourably. It can also include indirect discrimination, for example putting in place a rule or arrangement that is universal but puts certain protected characteristics at an unfair disadvantage. Finally, it can include harassment (behaviour that goes against people's dignity or creates an offensive environment in relation to a protected characteristic) and victimization (treating someone who complains about discrimination or harassment unfairly). Make sure that you read the pharmacy professional code of conduct before undertaking your placement or training.

Short placements arranged through your university

This section relates specifically to short placements arranged through your university, rather than summer posts and formal training posts, although the advice might be applicable to these other posts in some places.

Having agreed to host your placement, the organization will expect you to behave in the most professional manner, and in a way that does not interfere with the day-to-day running of their business or organization. You are reminded that as a pharmacy undergraduate undertaking a placement in a community, hospital, or other pharmacy setting, you are not only representing yourself as a future professional, but you are also representing your pharmacy school and university. It is really important, therefore, for you to adhere to certain standards of behaviour in order to promote a positive and professional image of yourself and your degree course. The purpose of attending your placement is to give you further insight into pharmacy, your chosen vocation. Therefore, having learnt the values of the NHS constitution, you should wholeheartedly apply them.

Remember that the pharmacists and pharmacy staff that will host your placement are giving their time to help you, so treat all staff with the respect they deserve. The world of pharmacy is relatively small and you will find that whichever branch of the profession you later join, you will inevitably come across pharmacists you have previously met, be it, for example, as work colleagues, at courses and conferences, or at specialist meetings, and so on. It really is best to start as you mean to go on.

Here are some suggestions to help you make a success of your pharmacy placement:

1. You could be required to make your own way to the placement and, what is more, travel costs might not be reimbursed by your university. Make sure that you find out about any travel advice and also arrangements that might be made for larger group visits.

2. Find out the start and finish time for your placement. Allow enough travel time so that you arrive with at least 15 minutes to spare. You can then make your way to the pharmacy and ask to see the contact pharmacist in good time.

3. Ask about lunch and break arrangements. You may be allowed 1 hour for lunch, but breaks may only be allowed at the discretion of the pharmacist.

4. You must not exceed 1 hour for lunch (and 15 minutes for tea breaks, where allowed). Where you are able to use a communal area (e.g. tearoom) for making tea/coffee, check to see if you should make a contribution for your drink, and keep the area clean and tidy.

5. Do not leave before the stated finish time of your placement (unless instructed to do so by the pharmacist).

6. Only take the necessary items to the placement with you. Do not take any valuables as there will be no guarantee that lockers will be available for safe storage of possessions.

7. Take with you a pen, a notepad, and any university-provided placements paperwork.

8. Your outfit should be smart and professional. For men this usually means smart trousers, shirt, and tie (although different rules may apply in the NHS, e.g. short sleeves and no tie). For women this means a smart dress, a smart top and skirt, or a smart top and trousers. Make sure that your hair is clean, tidy, and presentable.

9. Shoes should be smart, clean (and comfortable), and worn with appropriate socks/ hosiery. Trainers are not acceptable. Shoes should not be open-toed; sandals are not acceptable.

10. You should observe the uniform/dress code of the organization. This may include wearing an issued uniform.

11. Wear your university identity badge at all times if you are provided with one. You may also be issued with a visitor/student badge at the placement. Wear this as instructed and return at the end of the placement.

12. Switch off any mobile devices and do not use them at any time unless specifically instructed to do so (e.g. looking up a dose on the British National Formulary website using an iPad).

13. Familiarize yourself with social media guidelines if applicable (e.g. use of Twitter and Facebook) and make sure you adhere to them.

14. Do not consume food or drinks anywhere apart from designated areas (e.g. the tearoom/canteen). If unsure, ask your contact pharmacist. Similarly, chewing gum is not permitted. If you need to consume food for a medical reason or take medication in an undesignated area, please do so discreetly but make the pharmacist in charge aware beforehand.

15. Keep your behaviour professional and avoid non-professional discussions.

16. It is essential that you maintain the dignity of the patient at all times, through your own behaviour and appearance, and in any dealing that you may have with the patient (e.g. be discreet when discussing patient-related matters).

17. You must respect the patients' right to privacy. If a patient refuses your presence during their consultation with the pharmacist, accept courteously and re-join the pharmacist once he/she has moved on to the next patient.

18. Treat all information you receive in a confidential manner, be it relating to patients, the running of the business/premises, or any conversation that you may overhear.

19. At times, bear in mind that you might be asked to shadow the pharmacist. Do not obstruct his/her work (e.g. by asking unnecessary questions—instead, as much as possible, think about your questions and ask these at an appropriate interlude).

20. Work in a clean and tidy manner. Wash and dry your hands as appropriate (e.g. before and after visiting wards). In hospitals you may have to wash frequently and use an antiseptic hand rub between patients.

21. Do not forget to be polite and courteous in all your dealings with the staff at the placement and please do not leave without thanking the pharmacist (and other staff, if appropriate) for allowing you to shadow them for the duration of the placement.

22. Obtain the pharmacist's signature before you leave if you have been asked to do so.

Making the most of your placement or training post

Placements and training posts are of real value as they give you the chance to familiarize yourself with the practice of pharmacy and allow you to relate your learning to the workplace environment. Importantly, they also allow you to accrue experience to put in your personal/professional development portfolio and on your CV for future job applications and career progression.

During the course of your experience make notes of your activities where appropriate. Your experience may be very structured or you might find yourself merely shadowing a pharmacist or other members of staff with very little having been planned in advance. In any case, there are many examples of activities or behaviours that you can observe for your own learning. For example, you can keep an eye open for:

- a pharmaceutical calculation being carried out;
- a decision that needs the pharmacist's involvement;
- a patient being taught/counselled about their medicine(s);
- new terminology or abbreviations.

As you progress through your placement or post, you might form an opinion about a range of norms and practices:

- the role of the pharmacist as a provider of health care to patients;
- how the pharmacist fits into the health care team, including the role of support staff;
- how patient confidentiality is maintained.

We would advise that you make detailed notes (maintaining patient anonymity of course) so that you can later return and reflect on your observations. If the placement is a compulsory part of your course, it might well be formally assessed. For example, you might be asked to complete specific tasks or projects, write a report, write a reflective log or even use the learning in another course activity or assignment. If your placement is not linked to a formal assessment, or is not even a compulsory part of your degree course, it is still important for you to use the opportunity to demonstrate your learning in a personal/professional development portfolio. This will help you to call on your experience later to answer interview questions, for example.

To get you started, you could make a record of the following:

- the date(s) of your placement visit or training post;
- the name and address of the placement organization;
- the name and position of the contact person;
- your time of arrival, departure, and lunch/refreshment breaks;
- pharmacy operating hours;
- a log of the activities that you carried out/observed.

Reflecting on your practice placement or training post

One of the most important reasons for writing down an account of your activities during a placement or other post is to allow you to later reflect on your experience. Reflecting on your experience will allow you to learn more than you would by merely having the experience.

Although reflection is a very personal process it can be described as a form of thinking about an experience or a situation where you would gather all thoughts, feelings, and ideas in order to identify (for example) a new perspective, areas for change or improvement, or to note a summary of what has been learnt. Reflection allows you to draw generalizations or generate concepts that you would not develop through the experience alone. Without stopping and reflecting you might forget your placement experience relatively quickly, losing any potential it offered for further learning.

An example of a reflection from one of the authors' own 1-week community pharmacy placement during their pre-registration year is shown in Box 10.5.

On reading the example reflection in Box 10.5 you might have identified a number of features of this writing that are key to any process of reflection and reflective writing. Firstly, you will notice that the reflection is written in the first person; 'I', rather than the third person 'he/she' typically used in scientific writing. Secondly, you will notice that the author has explored and tried to provide an explanation of a particular event. This was not easy to do—the author had to be honest about their own past mistakes and the interactions they had with other people. At the same time, they have also tried to stand back from the experience and not take an overly defensive stance—they have had to set aside anxieties they had and try and present the experience in an honest way.

Although the description of the event is relatively thorough, the author has, in fact, left out many other details relating to their placement experience, making sure to leave room

Box 10.5   An example of a personal reflection on a placement experience

Reflection on a placement experience

In 1994, during a 1-week placement in a community pharmacy, I experienced what I considered to be a terrible example of practice. I had been sent to the pharmacy during my hospital pre-registration training year with the expectation that I would learn positively by shadowing the pharmacist and his pre-registration trainee. Yet it did not take me long to see that the pharmacist in charge was cavalier in his approach and I observed numerous examples of bad practice, including extemporaneous preparation of a tub of cream/ointment using 'marigold' gloves extracted from an outside toilet, leaving the actual pre-registration trainee in charge of dispensing and issuing dispensed items without a second check, placing patient-returned medication to stock, and so on. To make matters worse, a box fell on my head while I was standing in the dispensary—although it was not particularly heavy, it did surprise me!

I recall challenging the pharmacist about his actions, only to be told that the reality of community pharmacy was far from the ideals that I had been taught at university. Needless to say, I received no sympathy following the incident with the box—and there was no accident record book either. I found the pharmacist's dismissive tone patronizing.

At the time I thought it extremely ironic that I had been sent to that particular pharmacy to learn about community pharmacy! The following week I drafted a letter to the pharmacy regulator to report in absolute detail my experience and how, in my opinion, the pharmacist had breached the code of conduct during my placement. I showed the letter to my own pre-registration tutor, the chief pharmacist at my training hospital base. He questioned whether all of what I had listed in the letter was true and I replied that it certainly was and that I had no qualms whatsoever about posting the letter, which I did.

Now, more than 20 years on, I can reflect that my approach, although theoretically correct, was fuelled by the enthusiasm of youth and more inexperience! Nowadays, I would not dream of responding in that way. Perhaps the passage of time has dampened my sense of self-righteousness— it certainly felt very satisfying to turn the tables on that pharmacist for being in the wrong and for patronizing me! My understanding of people—how everyone has a viewpoint worth exploring—and the world of pharmacy—how small it is—and the need to develop and maintain one's reputation with colleagues would all lead me to a different response now. I would not draft any letter. Instead, I would take the lead from my own pre-registration tutor. If asked, I might suggest that we convene a meeting to establish the facts, hear the pharmacist's point of view, and develop an action plan for ensuring that inefficiencies which I identified are addressed.

for reflective insights, too. In their reflection, the author has tried to think about why they reacted in the way they did, for example. You will see that they have also tried to think about why the pharmacist was behaving in the way they were and what the author would do should a similar situation arise nowadays. We have written some general tips in Box 10.6 to help you with the process of reflecting on your own placement experience.

To truly learn from your practice placement or training post, you should take the process of reflection further by devising a continuing personal/professional development plan, which is explained in detail in Chapter 12. For now, note that following your reflection you should write down the detail of any points that you believe need further follow up. Think also about how your reflection might be of value for writing the personal statement in a future job application or for providing examples in a job interview.

Box 10.6 Tips for reflection on your placement or training experience

- Select one particular event or example relating to your placement or training post which challenged or puzzled you, or you thought was particularly successful.
- Explore and explain the detail of the example.
- Explore your interactions with others, and your feeling and reactions.
- Try to stand back from the situation and be as impartial as possible.
- Be critical of your own actions.
- Think of alternative explanations for the events.
- Acknowledge that your current viewpoint might change with time.
- Discuss the situation with others to explore a range of perspectives.
- Ask yourself:
    - Why did I respond in the way I did?
    - What was I thinking and feeling—did this influence me, and why?
    - What were the strengths and weaknesses of my actions (or lack of action)?
    - What was the other person/people thinking and feeling, what is the evidence for this?
    - How did my actions affect the situation?
    - How did the situation affect me?
    - What else could I have done?
    - What would I do in a similar situation?
- If relevant, think about how your experience compares with what you have read or theories that might explain what happened.
- Reflect on what might be the result of doing things differently.
- Has the experience changed your understanding of pharmacy?
- Can you link your reflections to the values in the NHS constitution?

 Key points

- Placements and training posts offer the opportunity to apply university learning in a pharmacy work setting.
- Placements and training posts can boost job prospects by allowing students to demonstrate experience in the field and insight about the profession.
- Sourcing summer and other work placements needs a methodical and persistent approach.
- Most employers will ask to see a CV or a completed application form and cover letter as part of formal job applications, and there are conventions for writing these.
- Employers want candidates to demonstrate good communication, teamwork and interpersonal skills, self-management, organizational skills, and the potential to learn and perform the specific job.
- A personal statement should clearly set out how the job description and person specification are met, with examples as appropriate.
- There are a number of standard interview questions, and some candidates read and prepare answers for these in advance of an interview.

- Values-based questions might be used to check whether personal values and behaviours of candidates match that of the NHS constitution.
- The values of the NHS constitution are: improving lives, respect and dignity, compassion, everyone counts, working together for patients, commitment to quality of care.
- A number of formalities might have to be met before visiting/working in pharmacy workplaces, including the DBS check and the occupational health check (work health assessment), which can take time to complete.
- Employees and employer/placement provider have a duty to take care of the health and safety of everyone within the workplace.
- Concerns about health and safety must be raised with a superior immediately.
- Accidents or work-related illnesses must be reported as soon as known.
- People's right to privacy must be fully respected at all times and patient identifiable information treated in a confidential manner.
- Any doubts about the processing of patient data should be raised with a person in authority at the workplace to obtain clarity.
- There should be no direct or indirect discrimination of people in a workplace.
- A record of activities or experiences within a placement or training post is a good starting point for reflection and further learning.
- Reflecting on an experience can help identify a new perspective, areas for change or improvement, or detail a summary of what has been learnt.
- There are a number of tips for reflecting and writing reflective pieces which can form the start of personal/professional development planning.

 Further reading and references

The Data Protection Act: https://www.gov.uk/data-protection/the-data-protection-act

Department of Health. Confidentiality: NHS Code of Practice. Leeds: Department of Health; 2003.

Department of Health. Confidentiality. *NHS Code of Practice* [downloadable PDF document]. Available from: https://www.gov.uk/government/uploads/system/uploads/attachment_data/file/200146/Confidentiality_-_NHS_Code_of_Practice.pdf [Accessed 25 October 2016].

Disclosure and Barring Service: https://www.gov.uk/disclosure-barring-service-check/overview

Employers: Preventing Discrimination: https://www.gov.uk/employer-preventing-discrimination/what-discrimination-is

European Agency for Safety and Health at Work. *Looking out for Work Hazards—Advice for Young People* [downloadable PDF document]. Available from: https://osha.europa.eu/en/tools-and-publications/publications/factsheets/66 [Accessed 25 October 2016].

National Careers Service: https://nationalcareersservice.direct.gov.uk/Pages/Home.aspx

NHS Employers. Values-based Recruitment [online]. Available from: http://www.nhsemployers.org/your-workforce/recruit/employer-led-recruitment/values-based-recruitment [Accessed 25 October 2016].

Watton P, Collings J, Moon J. *Reflective Writing. Guidance Notes for Students* [downloadable PDF document]. Available from: http://www.learnhigher.ac.uk/wp-content/uploads/Reflective_writing_The_Park_WattonCollingsMoon.pdf [Accessed 25 October 2016].

11 Understanding evidence-based practice

 Overview

Free access to huge amounts of information on the Internet has made patients more aware of health conditions, treatments, and tests than ever before. Consequently, it would not be unusual for a patient to come to you asking about a new treatment that they have read about. Therefore, you will need to be able to assess the accuracy of this information—the evidence base for it—and take into account that any clinical decision that is made in relation to the patient thereafter should involve consideration of their concerns, beliefs, and personal preferences.

Evidence-based practice (EBP) is commonly defined as the use of current best evidence to make decisions about the care of patients. In order to do this, you must consider clinical expertise, the best research evidence, and also patient preferences. It is important to remember that having the evidence itself does not make the decision for you. Rather, it provides you with the information needed to make the best clinical judgement for a particular patient. EBP also promotes an attitude of inquiry and gets you, as a health care professional, to think about why you are doing things in a certain way, how you could do things differently and more effectively, and reinforces your decisions and professional accountability.

This chapter complements Chapter 4, and describes the different types of evidence that health care practitioners have access to, how these can be interpreted, and how they can then be used in practice.

 Learning outcomes

You should be able to demonstrate knowledge and understanding of the following after working through this chapter:

- the hierarchy of evidence;
- different types of clinical studies and familiarity with common language used within clinical studies;
- evaluation of clinical evidence to answer a specific clinical question;
- statistical terms and concepts used in clinical studies.

The hierarchy of evidence

You may already be aware of the importance of using evidence from research and scientific studies to determine best practice. In general, the evidence found must be reliable, credible, and relevant to the reason you are looking for it. We test whether the evidence stands up to these criteria by *evaluating* it.

We can classify evidence as either primary or secondary, as discussed in Chapter 4. As a reminder, primary sources of evidence are those that report new data, results, or theories, and that were written by someone who directly participated in the research. Secondary sources of evidence are those that interpret and analyse primary sources of evidence. They are viewed by someone not directly involved in the original study; as such, they can be shaped by the author's interpretations, biases, and preconceptions. Exceptions to shaping by preconceived ideas are secondary sources such as systematic reviews or a meta-analysis.

Simply put, if the author is reporting first-hand observations then it is primary evidence, whereas if the author is conveying the experiences and opinions of others then the evidence is secondary.

There are also tertiary sources of literature, which summarize, abstract, or index the information derived from primary or secondary sources. These are useful to provide background information on your topic and include sources such as reference books and the British National Formulary. You may also come across 'grey literature' sources which are published in non-commercial form and may be difficult to obtain. Some of these may be peer reviewed and have some scientific merit. Examples include abstracts of conference papers, government reports, and policy statements.

Primary and secondary sources of evidence can be further classified according to a hierarchy: an evidence pyramid, as illustrated in Figure 11.1. At the bottom end of the pyramid are sources such as expert opinions; as you move up the pyramid the evidence becomes more robust, less biased, and more relevant to the clinical setting you are interested in.

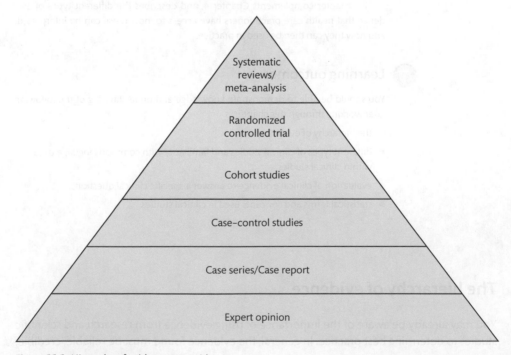

Figure 11.1 Hierarchy of evidence pyramid.

Let us now consider each of these sources of evidence.

Expert opinion is the lowest level of evidence as it relies on clinical experience only, not on the application of scientific rigour as seen with randomized, controlled clinical trials (RCTs).

Case series and case reports talk about individual patients, and do not include control groups or have any statistical validity. As such, these cannot be used to generalize to the wider population.

Case–control studies are different to case reports as they include a control group. Usually patients who have a specific condition are compared with people who do not have the condition. Those undertaking case–control studies typically look backwards (retrospectively) in patient histories to collect data.

Cohort studies are observational studies that take large populations of patients and follow them over a period of time. Comparisons of outcomes are made with a control group that was not exposed to the treatment or procedure under investigation.

RCTs are studies that involve methodologies that reduce the potential for bias and can include intervention or control groups for comparison. Bias is usually reduced by randomizing who is included in the study and through blinding (where the people conducting the trial do not know who is in the test, control, or intervention group). Trials are effectively carefully controlled experiments which can yield robust data about cause and effect of a particular treatment or procedure.

Systematic reviews are the most scientifically robust reviews and are more focused in terms of the clinical question being asked. The goal of a systematic review is to review high-quality studies in order to limit bias and produce reliable results to answer the question being asked. Thus, they involve a thorough literature search to identify studies of high quality (typically RCTs), analysis (ensuring the studies are methodologically and analytically robust, e.g. by meta-analysis), and then a summary of the overall evidence to address the question asked (Figure 11.2). They are therefore important in delivering EBP.

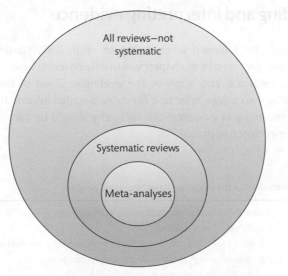

Figure 11.2 Systematic reviews and meta-analyses.

Adapted from Pai et al. (2004). © The National Medical Journal of India 2004.

> **Box** 11.1   Categories assigned to show the level of quality of a study
>
> | Level | Description |
> |---|---|
> | Ia | Well-designed meta-analysis of more than one randomized controlled trial |
> | Ib | Well-designed randomized, controlled study |
> | IIa | Well-designed controlled study without randomization |
> | IIb | Well-designed quasi-experimental study (i.e. lacking a key experimental component such as a control group, or randomization) |
> | III | Well-designed non-experimental studies, i.e. correlational and case studies |
> | IV | Expert committee report, consensus conference, clinical experience of respected authorities |

Meta-analysis can be used as part of a systematic review to synthesize the data from several studies into a single value or parameter. It is a statistical technique that is most often used to assess clinical effectiveness of interventions. The validity of the meta-analysis depends on the quality of the studies included in a systematic review. As the results from many trials are combined, the power of the meta-analysis increases, which then allows the detection of small, but clinically significant, effects. A mention of the statistical terms follows later in this chapter.

You may also see the hierarchy of evidence categorized as levels, which can be used to assign the level of quality of a study when undertaking a critical appraisal (Box 11.1). Assessing level of quality will be mentioned later.

In general, the hierarchy of evidence pyramid is a guide to the best level of study you can use to answer your clinical question. However, depending on the question you ask, you may not always find a RCT or systematic review, in which case you need to rely on clinical judgement and lower levels of evidence. We provide information about how you generate your clinical question and how you can go about critically appraising the evidence found later in the chapter.

Understanding and interpreting evidence

Several steps should be followed when trying to apply EBP, starting with the patient (Table 11.1). The next section of this chapter will briefly describe how to ask the right questions, acquire the evidence, and appraise the evidence. Some of this has already been discussed in Chapter 4 so please refer to it for more detailed information. We have briefly talked about the hierarchy of evidence; this hierarchy should be taken into account when thinking about the evidence appraisal.

Table 11.1 The steps involved in the evidence-based medicine process

The patient	Where the clinical problem or question arises from
The question	Clearly define your question
The evidence	Conduct a search to obtain the most relevant and highest level of evidence (Chapter 4)
Critical appraisal	Appraise the evidence for its validity and applicability
Apply the evidence	Use the findings to resolve the patient query

The question

Consider the following clinical scenario:

David is 43 years old and has a history of inflammatory bowel disease. He was diag-nosed with Crohn's disease in his early 20s and since then he has been in and out of hospital owing to severe exacerbations. David is managed on mesalazine, azathio-prine, and prednisolone, but feels this is not helping him much as his symptoms do not seem to be controlled and he wants to reduce his visits to the hospital.

During a recent holiday in the USA, David sees a television advert about a drug (Humira—adalimumab) that is meant to better target and control Crohn's disease. On his visit to pick up his prescription he asks you about this drug, but you are un-familiar with it and tell David that you will find out some more information and then get back to him.

How would you generate a clear clinical question in order for you to conduct a search for evidence?

PICO is a mnemonic that helps to identify the key search terms you might want to use:

- **P** is the patient or problem;
- **I** is the intervention, prognostic factor, or exposure;
- **C** is the comparison;
- **O** is the outcomes.

Table 11.2 outlines how to apply PICO.

If we apply PICO to David then this could look like:

P = Crohn's disease, male, 43 years old;

I = Humira/adalimumab;

C = none, standard care;

O = control of symptoms, reduced visits to the hospital.

Therefore the clinical question for David might be:

In male patients with Crohn's disease, is adalimumab effective in reducing the need for hospitalization?

Table 11.2 How to apply PICO

Patient or problem	What are the most important characteristics of your patient? Is it the disease? Is there anything else that might be relevant to the diagnosis or treatment, such as gender, age, or race?
Intervention	What is the main intervention, prognostic factor, or exposure you are considering? This could be a drug or surgery, or a test.
Comparison	What are you going to compare the intervention to (the alternative)? It could be another drug or test.
Outcomes	What are you trying to do for the patient, i.e. what is the measured outcome?

Acquiring the evidence

Once you have generated your clinical question, you can then think about your search strategy and how you will go about acquiring the evidence. Chapter 4 has already discussed the use of search terms, databases, and other sources of evidence in detail; we will refer back to this chapter where necessary. Remember that the practice of EBP requires practitioners to search primary literature to find their answers (although if there is a high-quality systematic review, then you may be justified in looking at this first). As such, choosing the best resource to search from is important.

If you are struggling with your literature search, a librarian or someone within your information services department can help you find research both in print and online, and can advise you on developing your search strategies. Also note that some databases and other resources provide you with direct access to online versions of the article, but this will be limited according to the subscriptions held by your place of work or institute. If you find you can't obtain a key article in electronic form, either because of no subscription or availability to download, don't be deterred from trying to obtain a paper copy: contact your library or even try emailing the corresponding author of the article. For a list of some of the databases and resources see Chapter 4.

Appraising the evidence

When appraising the primary literature that you have obtained, you should assess the quality of the study, which is pivotal when interpreting data, or when putting together a systematic review. There are various checklists available to assess quality of RCTs. These include the 5-point Jadad score (Jadad et al., 1996), which is used to assess the methodological quality of controlled trials and is commonly used in Cochrane reviews. Its short length and ease of use make it a common appraisal method. An international and widely used and recommended standard is the Consolidated Standards of Reporting Trials (CONSORT) statement, which uses a 25-item checklist. The items in the checklist focus on reporting how the trial was designed, analysed, and interpreted, but it does not technically rate the actual quality of a study, although it is often used in this way.

The following considerations for appraising the literature take into account the CONSORT checklist. However there is considerable overlap even among these different methods of evaluating trial quality.

Purpose of the research?	There should be a clear statement of the aims of the research. Is the research relevant to you?
Background to the research?	Previous research and the current state of knowledge, including a summary of key research articles, should be stated. If this information seems limited or biased then this will alter how the researcher contextualizes their findings.
Research method and study design?	This should be appropriate to answer your research question. Is it an RCT or case-control study? How were patients recruited (inclusion, exclusion criteria)? Who was under study? Does the population chosen represent those you are interested in? You can only draw conclusions about the population that you research. If it's a case report then the individual patient under study cannot represent all similar patients.

Who took part in the research?	Consider if the size and sampling procedure achieved a representative sample. Are any of your target population missing? Response rate is also crucial and can indicate whether the data collected is still representative.
Validity of results?	Validity should be looked at before an extensive analysis of the study is undertaken. If the study is not valid, the data may not be useful. Ask whether an intervention or control group was included and if these started with the same prognosis. Were the patients randomized? Was group allocation concealed, and to what extent was the study blinded? Was follow-up complete? Data are valid if the research measures what it intends to measure. These questions are further discussed below.
How are the results analysed?	If a study is quantitative in nature, then results are often analysed statistically. It is important to check that the statistical tests used are appropriate for the sample. If the study is qualitative then there should be an in-depth description of the analysis process. Typical tests include odds ratios, relative risk reduction, absolute risk reduction, numbers needed to treat, and *P*-values. These are further discussed below.
Interpretation of the results?	Are the interpretations based only on the results of the data generated in the study? Have any results been excluded, and were the limitations of the data collection method mentioned?
Validity of conclusions?	Are the conclusions clear and do they contextualize the findings appropriately?

As mentioned, the allocation of patients to the study group(s) must be done by *random* allocation. *Simple randomization* can include tossing a coin or using a sequence of random numbers from a statistical textbook. This is now often computer-generated using free software available online. Other methods of randomization include *permuted block randomization* and *stratified allocation*. Permuted block randomization is one way to achieve a balance of patients across treatment groups within a trial. For example, consider a controlled clinical trial with a treatment (A) and control (B) arm, with a sample size of 200 patients split equally between the two arms of the trial. You could decide to use 25 blocks of four patients (total 200 patients) and assign two patients to arm A and two to arm B. Using random selection, there would be six possible permutations in each block: AABB, BBAA, ABAB, BABA, ABBA, and BAAB. As long as enrolment into each block is completed, an equal number of patients in treatment and control arms is ensured.

Stratified randomization is used to ensure that equal numbers of participants with a characteristic thought to affect the response to the intervention will be allocated to each comparison group. For example, in a trial of women with osteoporosis, it may be important to have similar numbers of pre-menopausal and post-menopausal women in each comparison group. Stratified randomization could be used to allocate equal numbers of pre- and post-menopausal women to each treatment group.

By ensuring randomization you can help balance the groups for factors such as age, weight, socioeconomic status, and gender. Thus, randomization helps reduce bias by reducing the chance of over-representation of any one of these factors.

Ideally, randomization should be hidden (*concealed*) from the investigators in order to prevent them from predicting or changing the assignment of patients to the groups. The allocation sequence is not known to the investigators until the moment of assignment. If randomization has not been concealed, selection bias may occur. Concealment allocation can be done by using a centralized service or by the use of sealed envelopes.

In terms of the patients in the study groups, they should all be similar for all characteristics except whether or not they receive the intervention being tested. The article being critiqued should show this data, which are typically called the *baseline characteristics*.

Blinding means that the people involved in the study do not know which groups are the control or treatment groups. *Single blinding* usually refers to the patient being blinded to the treatment given but not the administering clinician. *Double blinding* is when neither the patient nor investigator knows which treatment the patient is randomized to. Placebo-controlled drug trials are usually double blind.

At the end of the study there should be the same number of patients in each group that was started with (*follow-up*). It is sometimes the case that a few patients drop out of a study for various reasons (adverse effect, death, refusing treatment), but all of these must be accounted for, otherwise there is the risk of the conclusions becoming invalid. Typically, good studies will have a follow-up of patients greater than 80%.

For an easy-to-understand worked example to help you start to critically analyse a RCT, the HealthKnowledge website (http://www.healthknowledge.org.uk) provides an e-learning tool, which provides you with a sample paper for you to review and then step-by-step guides, using the Critical Appraisal Skills Programme (CASP) methodology, to guide you through the critical appraisal process. CASP itself aims to help people develop the necessary skills to appraise scientific evidence and has produced checklists for both quantitative and qualitative research (including systematic reviews), which are freely and easily accessed on the Internet. We highly recommend that you look through the website and browse through the available checklists when undertaking your critical appraisal of a study.

Statistical terms

An important skill for critical evaluation of a research study is to be able to understand statistical terms. Table 11.3 lists the statistical terms most commonly used in clinical studies, with some worked examples later on in the chapter.

It should be noted that the descriptions of terms cited in Table 11.3 are just an overview and so lack the level of detail that you may need in choosing the appropriate statistical test and applying it. For example, sample size, power analysis, regression analysis, software packages for analysis (Statistical Package for the Social Sciences (SPSS), which can be used for descriptive analysis, regression, factor analysis, *t*-test, etc.), and other statistical terms are not mentioned here. However, a couple of simple examples to apply some of the terms in Table 11.3 to are provided below. It is important to bear in mind that poor use or poor interpretation of statistical tests can lead to erroneous outcomes and therefore ill-informed decision-making when it comes to patient care. Therefore, it is important to be able to appraise a study and know what the statistics mean. For more detailed information regarding statistics, the reader is referred to the *Oxford Handbook of Medical Statistics* or *Statistical Evidence in Medical Trials* (both published by Oxford University Press).

Applying the statistical terms

Whenever we look at RCTs to determine whether a treatment is of benefit to the patient, we also want to see what the frequency of poor or undesired outcomes of an intervention in the group being treated compared with those who were not treated is. This can, in the first instance, be done by looking at the percentage of undesired outcomes in the intervention

Table 11.3 Statistical terms used for analysis of clinical data

Statistical term	What does this tell us?
P-value	The probability that an observed difference occurred by chance. By convention, if the P-value is less than 1 in 20 ($P < 0.05$) then the result is regarded as being 'statistically significant'. So the smaller the P-value the less likely the data were by chance and more likely due to the intervention under investigation
Confidence intervals (CIs)	The CI indicates the level of uncertainty around the measure of effect. In other words, it is the range of values within which the true value lies. The narrower the range, the more reliable the results. If the CIs of two interventions overlap then the trial has failed to show a difference between the two. In most cases 95% CIs are used, which means that you can be 95% sure that the true value lies between the figures quoted
Event rate (ER)	The proportion of patients in a group in whom the event is observed. For example, if we have 100 patients, and the event is observed in 50, the ER is 0.5 or 50%. When linking event rates to the intervention, i.e. control and experimental groups, then you will commonly see control ER (CER) and experimental ER (EER) referred to. Sometimes, the ER is also referred to as the absolute risk (AR)
Absolute risk reduction (ARR)	Sometimes referred to as the risk difference (RD), it is the arithmetic difference between the ER in the experimental and control groups (ARR = CER − EER). It refers to the change in the risk of an outcome of a given intervention in relation to a comparison intervention, or, put another way, whether there is a decrease in a bad/undesired event as a result of the intervention
Relative risk (RR)	How many times more likely it is that an event will occur in the intervention group relative to the control group (RR = EER ÷ CER). For example, a RR of 0.80 means that the intervention group had a 20% reduced risk of an event compared with those in the control group. An RR of < 1 is good if you want less of something (e.g. pregnancy or heart attack); an RR > 1 is good if you want more of something (women using contraceptives or eating healthier)
Relative risk reduction (RRR)	The proportional reduction in risk between the rates of events in the experimental and control groups (RRR = (CER − EER) ÷ CER or more simply ARR ÷ CER). RRR is often a larger number than the ARR
Odds ratio (OR)	The OR is a relative measure of effect, which allows the comparison of the experimental group relative to the control group. The odds of an event (primary outcome) occurring is the number of times an event (primary outcome) will happen divided by the number of times it won't happen. For example, if in a group of 100 patients treated with a painkiller, 35 got appreciable pain relief and 65 patients didn't, then the odds for patients getting pain relief over those not having any benefit would be 35 ÷ 65 = 0.54. If in the control group (no painkiller) the odds are 1 (pain relief) divided by 99 (no pain relief), which = 0.01, then the OR will be 0.54 ÷ 0.01 = 54. In general, the smaller the OR, the more effective the intervention is at reducing that primary outcome compared to control. The larger the OR, the less effective the intervention, and if OR is 1, there is no difference between the groups
Number needed to treat (NNT)	The number of patients who would need to be treated in order to prevent one bad outcome or produce one good outcome. NNT is calculated by dividing 1 by ARR.

versus the control group. However, without knowing more about the undesired outcomes (usually adverse effects) all you can say is that the incidence of the undesired outcome in one of the study groups/arms is reduced.

For example, let's consider David, the patient with Crohn's disease we mentioned earlier. You find a RCT that shows that for patients similar in baseline characteristics to David, the percentage of those patients who took Humira and developed adverse effects such as infections, nausea, and abdominal pain was 15% compared with 5% in the control group. Is this 10% difference meaningful for patients like David? This is where you need to consider the risk of treatment versus no treatment, where risk is the probability of an undesired outcome occurring. So we look at the definitions of relative risk (RR), absolute risk reduction (ARR), number needed to treat (NNT), and relative risk reduction (RRR) and apply these to David's example.

The ARR is –10% (5% – 15% = –10% or –0.1). This means that, if 100 patients with Crohn's disease were treated, 10 would go on to *develop* adverse effects. If the numbers were reversed and the trial showed that 15% in the control group experienced adverse effects versus 5% in those taking the drug, then we would say that 10 patients would be *prevented* from getting an undesired outcome. So, in the context of the example, adding Humira will lead to 10% of patients developing adverse effects.

Another way of expressing the ARR is the number needed to treat (NNT). If 10 out of 100 patients with Crohn's disease experience adverse effects from treatment, the NNT is 10 (1 ÷ 0.1 = 10), which means that you will need to treat 10 people for 1 person like David to get an adverse effect. Health policy-makers need to weigh this against cost and treatment effects because it might not be seen as cost-effective if more than 1 out of every 10 patients treated experiences adverse effects and discontinues treatment.

As mentioned in Table 11.3, the RR of an undesired outcome in a group given the intervention is a proportional measure that estimates the size of the effect of a treatment compared with other interventions or no treatment at all. It is the proportion of undesired outcomes in the intervention group divided by the proportion of undesired outcomes in the control group. For David's example, the RR is 3 (15% ÷ 5% = 3). So as the RR > 1, then the risk of the adverse effects is increased by the treatment. In this case we can say that the chance of adverse effects in patients taking Humira is three times more likely to occur with treatment than without it.

RRR, which tells you by how much the treatment reduces the risk of undesired outcomes in comparison with the control group who did not have the treatment, would be –2 (ARR ÷ CER = –10 ÷ 5 = –2). This means there is actually a risk increase (when converted to a percentage = 200%) as opposed to a risk reduction when compared with the control group. So in the context of the example, adding Humira increases the event rate of an undesired outcome occurring by 200%.

So you can see that, in this case, you could argue that the risk of adverse effects is high when taking the treatment, whichever statistical test you decide to use to calculate risk (whether it is ARR or RRR), which may be something you would want to consider before starting David on the new treatment. However, what we haven't considered yet is the statistics regarding the positive outcomes of treatment (e.g. reduced symptoms or increased lifespan). You would follow the same calculations as above and then make an evidence-based judgement on whether you think the benefit of treatment outweighs the risk.

One point of note is that clinical significance is not the same as statistical significance. For a finding to be clinically important a substantial change in an outcome is looked for. Statistical significance depends on the number of observations that have been made. In essence, clinical significance has less to do with statistics and more to do with judgement. It often depends on the magnitude of the effect being studied. For example, a study of a sufficient size might find that a new antidiabetic drug lowers glycated haemoglobin (HbA1c) levels by 1 mmol/mol, on average, compared with metformin; this difference might be shown to be statistically significant ($P < 0.05$). However, in practice this difference in HbA1c levels may not be large enough to justify the use of the new drug. In other words, it is clinically insignificant.

Once you have done your critical review you need to look back at your initial question and see how you can apply your findings to your patient. It is worth reminding yourself of the following questions:

- Were the study patients similar to my population of interest?
- Are the likely treatment benefits worth the potential harm?
- Are the likely treatment benefits worth the potential costs?

Integrating evidence with practice

One way that EBP can help get the best available evidence into clinical practice is by way of guidelines. Clinical guidelines provide a professional consensus on a particular disease and its treatment, and are based on clinical experience, professional expertise, and a strong evidence base (RCTs, systematic reviews, and meta-analyses). Guidelines can cover any aspect of a disease and may include recommendations about providing information and advice to patients, prevention, diagnosis, treatment, and long-term management. As a result, guidelines are used heavily in health care. The main source of guidelines with which most people are familiar are those issued by the National Institute for Health and Care Excellence (NICE), which is an independent organization responsible for providing national guidance. Its guidelines are recommendations, based on the best available evidence from a range of different sources. Other sources of clinical guidelines are the Scottish Intercollegiate Guidelines Network (SIGN) and some professional organizations and Royal Colleges.

Guideline development and use thus depends on the strength of recommendation, which is usually categorized as A–D and linked to the level of evidence described earlier in Box 11.1:

A—Directly based on level I evidence

B—Directly based on level II evidence or extrapolated recommendation from level I evidence

C—Directly based on level III evidence or extrapolated recommendation from level I or II evidence

D—Directly based on level IV evidence or extrapolated recommendation from level I, II, or III evidence

For patients, the use of guidelines by health care professionals means that they should have improved health outcomes and a consistency of care. For health care professionals, guidelines are beneficial because up-to-date information is provided, they can help provide a consistency of care, they call to attention ineffective or dangerous practices, highlight interventions that are unsupported by evidence, they support quality improvement activities such as audits, and increase the use of critical-care pathways. In essence, sticking to the clinical guidelines proves commitment to excellence and quality. However, just be aware that not all guidelines are evidence-based (there are many that are not published by NICE), or they may be out of date (so check the published date and when it is due for an update), or simply that there is no clinical evidence or guideline for the use of a particular drug. Therefore, in these cases it is important to use your scientific, clinical, and professional judgement when making decisions about treatment.

Barriers to evidence-based practice

EBP is not without its criticisms and drawbacks. These include the following:

- it can be time consuming to undertake;
- research within the field of investigation may be limited, making it difficult to provide the evidence to base practice upon;
- there will never be answers to every possible clinical question;
- professional practice is forever changing, and is complex and evolving, which can make the information acquired no longer relevant;
- some authors think EBP relies heavily on quantitative methods instead of qualitative research, which is important in understanding what people believe or perceive health to be and how they go about managing their own health and making decisions;
- the nature of evidence is a matter of debate, with some questioning whether research should be the only source of this evidence.

The reservations associated with employing EBP do not prevent its use as it is a widely adopted approach and is here to stay. You as a future health care professional will be relying heavily on this in order to provide the best care for your patients.

 ## Real-practice examples

Example 1

Consider a double-blinded RCT studying drug X (intervention) versus placebo (P) with the aim of reducing the risk of getting cancer over 2 years. Each group contains 12,000 volunteers. The number of incidents of cancer in the drug X group is 1500 and the number in the P group is 2000.

If we want to know what the event rate (ER) is for each group, then

ER in X group = 1500/12000 = 0.125 or 12.5%
ER in P group = 2000/12000 = 0.167 or 16.7%
ARR = 0.167 − 0.125 = 0.042 or 4.2%

This means that 4.2% of the population will not develop cancer when treated with drug X.

For the RRR, then
RRR = ARR ÷ ER in P group = 0.042/0.167 = 0.251 or 25.1%

which means that 25% fewer patients develop cancer when treated with drug X.

Looking at the NNT, which describes the number of patients that we need to treat with drug X for 2 years to prevent one patient getting cancer, then
NNT = 1/ARR
NNT = 1/0.042 = 23.81

This means that 23 patients need to be treated with drug X for 2 years to prevent one patient getting cancer, which is a large number and so from a cost-effectiveness point of view may not be a useful drug if reducing the risk of cancer is considered its main advantage.

Looking at the OR, then the odds of getting cancer = number of times cancer occurs divided by number of times it doesn't occur, which is

The odds in X group = 1500/10500 = 0.143
The odds in group P = 2000/10000 = 0.2
OR = 0.143/0.2 = 0.715

So this value of OR means that drug X is better than placebo at reducing the risk of getting cancer.

Example 2

Mr Jones is 65 years old and was admitted to hospital after having several attacks of severe chest pain, which occurred even when he was not doing anything strenuous. He was first given an aspirin tablet and then given morphine. His cardiac enzymes were elevated and his electrocardiogram was normal. He was put on oxygen and a glyceryl trinitrate (GTN) drip for 24 hours, and also given clopidogrel and a low molecular weight heparin. The diagnosis was a non-ST-segment elevated myocardial infarction (NSTEMI).

Mr Jones has a past medical history of angina for which he was taking sublingual GTN, aspirin, simvastatin, and atenolol. The consultant looking after Mr Jones wanted him to start on a new drug he had heard about and came to speak to you about whether you thought it would be effective in treating Mr Jones' angina.

You undertake a literature search and find a double-blinded RCT studying the drug mentioned by the consultant (drug X) versus no drug X (control group (C)) on the risk of cardiovascular events over 3 years. A large population size was selected and randomized to each group. The baseline characteristics included both men and women, aged between 55 and 75 years of age, with a previous history of angina and no other comorbidities. All the patients included in the study had received standard care. All patients were accounted for; none dropped out of the trial. Based on this RCT would you recommend Mr Jones receive drug X and why?

Outcome	Control (n = 10,000)	Drug X (n = 10,000)	95% CI	P-value
	No. of patients with event	No. of patients with event		
Primary outcome	3380	2339	0.95 (0.86–1.05)	0.03
Death	400	375		
Heart failure	775	770		
Myocardial infarction	2000	1000		
Unstable angina	80	75		
Stroke	110	101		
Ventricular arrhythmia	15	18		

CI, confidence interval.

You are interested in the number of patients at risk of having a myocardial infarction (MI).

1. What is the ER for the control (no drug X) and intervention (drug X) groups?

2. What is the ARR for having an MI and what does this tell you?

3. What is the RRR?

4. Calculate the OR for getting an MI. What does this tell you?

5. Determine the NNT for the MI outcome. What does this mean?

Key points

- EBP is the use of current best evidence to make decisions about the care of patients. Evidence found must be reliable, credible, and relevant to the reason you are looking for it.

- There is a hierarchy of evidence which you must consider when using research studies to inform best practice. Systematic reviews are considered the most scientifically robust type of review of research.

- Being able to appraise evidence is an essential skill when undertaking EBP. For example, use of the CASP methodology provides useful checklists for how to appraise difference sources of evidence.

- You must become familiar with terminology used, and their meaning, when describing research methodology and results (statistical terms).

- Clinical guidelines are a good source for determining the best course of treatment for a patient.

- However, there may be some instances when there will not be any clinical evidence on the use of a drug—what should you do then? This is when the use of your scientific skills and knowledge that are unique to pharmacists (chemistry, pharmaceutics, pharmacology) become key.

 References and further reading

Bland M. An Introduction to Medical Statistics. 4th ed. Oxford: Oxford University Press; 2015.

The *BMJ. How to Read a Paper* [online]. Available from: http://www.bmj.com/about-bmj/resources-readers/publications/how-read-paper [Accessed 23 January 2016].

Consolidated Standards of Reporting Trials (CONSORT): http://www.consort-statement.org

Critical Appraisal Skills Programme (CASP): http://www.casp-uk.net

Enhancing the QUAlity and Transparency Of health Research (EQUATOR) : http://www.equator-network.org

HealthKnowledge. *Video Courses* [online]. Available from: http://www.healthknowledge.org.uk/interactive-learning [Accessed 23 January 2016].

Jadad AR, Moore RA, Carroll D, Jenkinson C, Reynolds DJM, Gavaghan DJ, et al. Assessing the Quality of Reports of Randomized Clinical Trials: Is Blinding Necessary? Control Clin Trials. 1996; 17(1):1–12.

National Elf Service. Evidence-based Practice [online]. Available from: http://www.nationalelfservice.net/evidence-based-practice [Accessed 23 January 2016].

National Institute for Health and Care Excellence (NICE): https://www.nice.org.uk/

Pai M, McCulloch M, Gorman JD, Pai N, Enanoria W, Kennedy G, et al. Systematic Reviews and Meta-analyses: An Illustrated, Step-By-Step Guide. Natl Med J India. 2004; 17(2):86–95.

Peacock J, Peacock P. Oxford Handbook of Medical Statistics. Oxford: Oxford University Press; 2010.

Schardt C, Mayer J. *An Introduction to the Principles of Evidence-based Practice* [downloadable PDF document]. Available from: http://www.hsl.unc.edu/services/tutorials/ebm/ebp_tutorial.pdf [Accessed 25 October 2016].

Simon SD. Statistical Evidence in Medical Trials. What do the Data Really Tell Us? Oxford: Oxford University Press; 2006.

Students 4 Best Evidence : http://www.students4bestevidence.net/

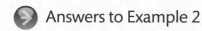 Answers to Example 2

1. What is the ER for the control (no drug X) and intervention (drug X) groups?

   A. ER in X group = 1000/10000 = 0.1 or 10%

   ER in C group = 2000/10000 = 0.2 or 20%

2. What is the ARR for having an MI and what does this tell you?

   A. The ARR = 0.2 – 0.1 = 0.1 or 10%, which means 10% of the population will not develop an MI when treated with drug X.

3. What is the RRR?

   A. RRR is the ARR divided by the ER in the control group = (10/20) = 0.5 or 50%, which means that 50% fewer people will develop an MI when treated with drug X.

4. Calculate the OR for getting an MI. What does this tell you?

   A. The odds in drug X group = 1000/9000 = 0.11

   The odds in group C = 2000/8000 = 0.25

   Therefore the OR = 0.11/0.25 = 0.44. As this value is < 1 (remember the smaller the value, the more effective the intervention is at reducing that primary outcome) then this means that having the intervention (taking drug X) reduces the risk of having an MI (by 66%) compared with not taking the drug.

5. Determine the number needed to treat (NNT) for the MI outcome. What does this mean?

   A. NNT is calculated as 1 divided by ARR = 1/0.1 = 10. This means that 10 patients need to be treated with drug X for 3 years to prevent one MI. Put another way, the clinician would need to treat 10 patients with drug X to achieve one additional patient with a favourable outcome (no MI).

   The study is a double-blind RCT, which means it has a high level of evidence and would be considered of good quality (there is a control group, the sample size is large, randomization was used). Looking at the baseline characteristics of the study, Mr Jones seems to fit the inclusion criteria and so the results would be applicable to him. The data would seem valid as no patient dropped out of the study. Statistical analysis of the data shows that there is benefit in taking drug X and it does not increase the risk of an MI. In addition, the CI is in a narrow range and $P < 0.05$. Therefore, you could recommend to the consultant that drug X may be suitable for Mr Jones based on these trial data.

12 Continuing professional development

 Overview

This chapter is about continuing professional development, or CPD. This topic will be important to you now, as a student, and in the future, as a health care professional. During this chapter, we will look at what the CPD process is, how to identify CPD opportunities, and how to construct effective CPD records. As a student, being able to reflect on your knowledge and skills, identify strengths and weaknesses, and take action to improve will help you to make the most of your studies and reach your full potential. In the future, it is likely that you will need to provide evidence of your CPD to the pharmacy regulator or your employer, so learning how to carry out effective CPD now will be useful for your future career.

 Learning outcomes

You should be able to demonstrate knowledge and understanding of the following after working through this chapter:

- what CPD is, and its importance;
- the stages of the CPD cycle;
- how to construct a CPD record.

What is continuing professional development?

In a nutshell, CPD is everything that we do that allows us to grow and develop as health care professionals, expanding and honing our knowledge, skills, and behaviours. It is a continuous and lifelong process in which individuals take responsibility for their own development, reflecting on their strengths and weaknesses, and taking action to address any learning needs that they identify. In 2003, the Department of Health published a report that defined CPD as 'a wide range of learning activities through which professionals maintain and develop throughout their career to ensure that they retain their capacity to practise safely, effectively and legally within their evolving scope of practice'. (This report was entitled the 'Allied Health Professions Project: Demonstrating Competence Through Continuing Professional Development'. Full details are given in the Further Reading and References section.)

For pharmacists, CPD is a professional responsibility and regulatory requirement, ensuring that we remain up to date in our knowledge and skills, and safe in our practice. Ultimately, the focus of CPD for health care professionals is optimizing patient care.

The continuing professional development process

Everyone learns in different ways and there are different models of CPD. However, the process that is most commonly referred to within pharmacy is the CPD cycle, as shown in Figure 12.1. As you can see in Figure 12.1, there is no set starting point in the CPD cycle. This is because learning can occur in different ways—sometimes you might identify a gap in your knowledge while thinking back, or 'reflecting', on how you have performed in a certain task, whereas at other times something unexpected might occur which allows you to learn something. The point at which you start in the cycle is less important than what you actually learn and how you apply your learning.

The stages of the continuing professional development cycle

Let's now consider each of the stages shown in Figure 12.1 in more detail.

Reflection

Although one can start anywhere in the CPD cycle, reflection is often thought of as the first step in a full CPD cycle. It is where you think about your knowledge and skills, what you do well, and where you might need to improve. This reflection may be prompted by a range of different factors:

- Critical incidents—an event in which you feel you might have acted in a different way, or achieved more. This may be an assessment in which you feel you could have performed better, or a situation that occurs while on placement. This may prompt you to identify knowledge, behaviour, or a skill that you could develop.

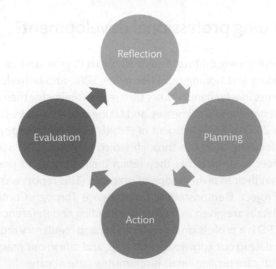

Figure 12.1 The continuing professional development cycle.

- Talking to others—speaking with your peers or other colleagues can be a really useful way of identifying an area in which you could improve.

- Feedback from others—this could be feedback from a peer, a colleague or a lecturer, an appraisal with a manager while on placement, or feedback from a patient that you have interacted with. This doesn't have to be negative feedback—receiving positive comments about your performance can often highlight areas in which you can 'step up' to the next level.

- Personal interest—this might be a topic that you are interested in learning more about for your own personal interest, or perhaps you are going to be taking on summer vacation work and need to develop your knowledge and skills in order to be able to perform that role effectively.

Personal development planning can be a useful tool to support the CPD process, encouraging you to reflect on your own performance and achievements, identify strengths and areas for improvement, and plan your personal, educational, and career development.

Another tool that you might find useful to help guide your CPD, particularly once qualified, is the Royal Pharmaceutical Society's Foundation Pharmacy Framework (see Further Reading and References section for full details). This framework describes a set of competencies and behaviours and can be used to assess yourself and identify learning gaps as you develop through your early career.

The ability to reflect is important for health care professionals; we can't rely on others to identify our learning needs and must be able to spot areas in which we can improve in order to provide the best quality of patient care possible. Because of the importance of reflection, you are likely to be expected to ensure that a proportion of your CPD starts at this stage of the cycle, so don't be tempted to skip this step in favour of entries that are quicker to complete!

Planning

This stage will normally be linked to a period of reflection: you've identified something that you need to develop and now need to think about how you will go about that. Within this stage you will need to consider the timescale within which you need to complete the learning, the importance of obtaining the particular knowledge or skill, and identify possible ways in which you can achieve it. Later in the chapter we will look at different sources of learning that can be used.

Action

So, you have identified what you need to learn and have thought about how you might achieve that. The action stage is the point at which you actually carry out the learning and describe what you have learnt.

Evaluation

This is an important part of the cycle—you should always evaluate what you have done. Did you achieve what you intended to? How have you/others actually benefitted from what you have learnt? How have you applied your learning? If you didn't achieve what you had hoped to, this is the point at which you think about why that might be and what you need to do next.

Identifying relevant continuing professional development

The topics that you choose for your CPD should be personal to you—you will have your own areas of strength and those needing development, and your CPD should reflect that. There is no 'right or wrong' topic for CPD—the important thing is that it is relevant to what you are, or will be, doing (so, in the context of this book, relevant to your studies or the practice of pharmacy). If you are completing CPD entries as part of an assessment (e.g. a piece of coursework) then you will need to ensure that you follow any instructions that you have been given in your assessment brief.

Ideally, topics for learning should be those for which you can demonstrate a benefit. This may be by applying them to a situation in which you are caring for a patient, and can also be in relation to other aspects of your role as a student or practitioner. If you have identified a topic but, as part of your planning process, decide that it is of low importance to you or others, you should think about whether it is appropriate to use it as the basis of a CPD entry.

Let's now consider some examples of CPD topics.

Clinical topic—management of hay fever

Sue is a second-year pharmacy student undertaking a 4-week community pharmacy summer placement. On her first day she was asked to spend some time on the medicines counter, observing one of the counter assistants. She noticed that there was a promotion of hay fever treatments at the pharmacy and realized that she did not know what all of the different products were. She thought that this was something that would be important to know about, as many people suffer from hay fever during the summer and she wanted to be able to advise customers on the most appropriate treatment for them. She decided that she would complete a CPD cycle in order to improve her knowledge of this topic.

Working with others—negotiation skills

Nancy is a community pharmacist. The pharmacy that she works in provides supplies of medicines to residents of a local nursing home and she is hoping to increase the scope of the service that they provide. She has always found negotiating difficult to do—it makes her feel uncomfortable and she feels that she never achieves the outcomes that she is hoping for. She therefore decides that it would be helpful to learn about some techniques that would help her to develop her negotiation skills. She decides to complete a CPD cycle in order to improve her skills in this area.

Working with patients—consultation skills

Tom is a first-year pharmacy student. On a recent visit to a local hospital he had the chance to talk to a patient about their medicines. He found the experience interesting but felt that he could have performed better in discussing the patient's medicines. He has been learning about communication and consultation skills as part of his course, and has also carried out some role plays with his friends in workshops. He had thought that he had been doing well in the role plays but found the consultation with a 'real' patient quite different. He would like to improve his consultation skills so that when he has the opportunity to speak to a patient in his next placement, he feels more confident in speaking with them. He decides to complete a CPD cycle to improve his skills in this area.

Administrative skills—working with computers

Rav is a hospital pharmacist who has just started a new job as a specialist cancer pharmacist. Part of this new role is to provide reports on the hospital's expenditure on cancer treatments. As he is new to the hospital, he is unfamiliar with the pharmacy computer system and is not able to run the reports that he needs to be able to calculate the expenditure on dispensed medicines. He decides to complete a CPD cycle to improve his knowledge of this topic and enable him to successfully produce the required reports.

Effective organizational performance—knowing the structure of the organization for which you work

Amareen has been working in the pharmaceutical industry for 11 months. There was recently an issue with the manufacture of one of the company's new medicinal products, which required her to liaise with a variety of staff from other sections in the company in order to resolve the problem. Thinking back on how she handled the problem, she realized that her knowledge of who to speak to in the other sections was not as good as it should be: she wasn't familiar with who the appropriate specialists were, which meant that it took her longer to resolve the problem than it might otherwise have done. She decides to complete a CPD cycle to improve her knowledge of how the organization is structured and the details of staff with relevant responsibilities.

Conducting continuing professional development

So, you have identified something that you need to learn or develop. What next? The next step is to look at the specific detail of what you would like to learn or develop (your learning objective), after which you need to think about how you will achieve this.

The learning objective

Let's consider the first scenario given above—the treatment of hay fever. Although it might, at first, seem a clear and specific topic to learn about, it actually could be interpreted in many different ways. For example, we might be referring to the medicines available without prescription for the treatment of hay fever in a certain patient group (e.g. children), how to select the most appropriate treatment for a patient with existing medical conditions, the legal restrictions that apply to certain hay fever treatments on sale to the public (e.g. corticosteroid nasal sprays), or the usual doses for all commonly available hay fever treatments. It is therefore important to think about the level of detail required when setting your learning objective. For example, 'I would like to learn the non-prescription pharmacological treatment options available for hay fever in adults and the recommended doses of each'. When thinking about writing objectives, the 'SMART' acronym is often used to support their effective preparation:

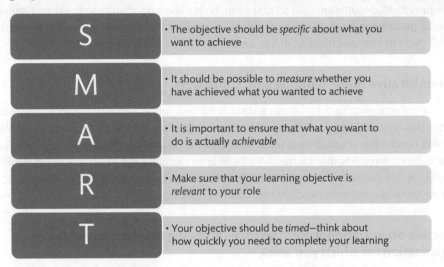

S	• The objective should be *specific* about what you want to achieve
M	• It should be possible to *measure* whether you have achieved what you wanted to achieve
A	• It is important to ensure that what you want to do is actually *achievable*
R	• Make sure that your learning objective is *relevant* to your role
T	• Your objective should be *timed*—think about how quickly you need to complete your learning

An example of a SMART objective might be: 'By the end of the month I would like to be able to use correctly the Harvard referencing system when writing an essay'. This objective is *specific*, as it clearly identifies what needs to be achieved (being able to reference using Harvard) and in what context (when writing an essay); it is *measurable*, as it can easily be assessed whether or not an essay has been correctly referenced; it is *achievable* within the timeframe given; it is *relevant* (assuming that your university uses the Harvard system); and it has a clear *timescale*.

When planning what you will do to learn what you want to learn, you should think about a range of different ways in which you might achieve this and the timescale in which you need to complete the learning. You should generally avoid using textbooks as the sole source of information, as they may become 'out of date' and not reflect current practice. For many people, reading a book is not a very effective way of learning, making it important to consider what options are available and which of these best suit you and what you want to learn. Some sources of learning include:

- reading a textbook or journal article;
- observing a more experienced student or practitioner;
- discussing with a peer or colleague;
- attending a lecture, workshop, or seminar;
- completing an e-learning package;
- attending a meeting.

You do not necessarily need to undertake all of the options that you think about in the planning stage—thinking about the advantages and disadvantages of each method of learning will help you to decide which are most appropriate to what you want to achieve. Think about the topic you are hoping to cover; a textbook would be a good starting place for learning about physiology, whereas observing an experienced pharmacist is likely to be much more useful when learning how to take a medication history from a patient. Remember to bear in mind whether the approaches that you are considering are sensible in terms of the time you have available. You may wish to attend a training course on the subject you have chosen; however, if this is not available until 6 months' time and you need to complete your learning in 3 weeks, this is clearly not going to be an appropriate method for this particular piece of learning. You should also consider how you learn best and choose methods which you find most useful. Some people enjoy reading articles, whereas others find that they learn more effectively through discussion with others.

Once you have completed the learning activities that you have selected, the final step is to think about what you have learnt and its impact on you and your practice.

Noting outcomes from continuing professional development

While you will probably agree with the importance of identifying what knowledge and skills you need to develop, and undertaking activities to address these, you may not be so convinced by the need to then evaluate and record what you have done.

The evaluation stage is crucial because it encourages you to think about what you have done, what you have gained from it, and whether you need to take any further action to achieve fully what you originally set out to achieve. Even a small piece of learning can lead to an important change in practice or behaviour that is carried forward throughout your career. When evaluating your learning, you may find it helpful to consider how you have actually applied what you have learnt—perhaps in relation to an interaction you have had with a patient during a placement or work experience, or perhaps in relation to your degree programme.

Making records will help you in this process of evaluation and further reflection, and also serve as evidence to others of the learning that you are undertaking—this will be important as part of demonstrating ongoing competence in your future career.

Constructing continuing professional development records

Let us now take a look at how to write a CPD record—what to include and things to think about when constructing them. Just as there are many ways in which we can approach our learning and development, there are a variety of ways in which CPD can be recorded; your university may specify its own format that you should use. We will use the format recommended by the pharmacy regulator, the General Pharmaceutical Council (GPhC), to provide the structure of this section, but the general principles of a good CPD record will apply to whatever format you use. Figure 12.2 shows an example layout of a CPD record adapted from the GPhC document for use in a university setting.

Where do I start?

It can sometimes be difficult to identify the stage of the CPD cycle at which to start your entry. Figure 12.3 provides some examples, which will hopefully help you to decide.

In the example of 'starting at reflection', the student is thinking about their own knowledge and skills, and identifying something that they would like to change or develop to help them to improve their practice for the future; in this case, in a placement that they are soon to undertake.

In the 'starting at planning' example, the student has not carried out the process of reflection—they are not attending the seminar because of a specific learning need that they have

LEARNING THAT STARTS AT REFLECTION

Name of entry _____   Date learning need identified _ _ / _ _ / 20 _ _

REFLECTION

What do you want to learn?

What you need to learn may be new knowledge, skills, or a new attitude – anything which will help you to change your practice for the better. You should make it as specific as possible.

How did you identify what you needed to learn?

Explain how you chose what to learn.

How is this learning relevant to the safe and effective practice of pharmacy and your own job role/ future career as a pharmacist?

PLANNING

When will you need to have achieved this learning?   _ _ / _ _ / 20 _ _

Putting an estimated date may help you to set priorities for your learning. Be as specific as possible, but don't worry if the date is just an approximation.

Why is this learning important to you and your practice?

Write a brief description of how this learning will affect you and your customers/patients. If you don't think that your learning will have a significant impact on anyone, you might want to consider why you are undertaking and recording this learning.

What might you need to do in order to achieve this learning?

It is important for you to consider a range of options for achieving your learning. Aim to list a few different options (e.g. attend workshops, reading articles or training packs, or talking to colleagues). Outline what you think are the advantages and disadvantages of each option. You may not choose to complete all the options that you've listed, but it is important that you have considered them.

Option	Description of what you plan to do	Advantages	Disadvantages	Select (√ or x)
1				
2				
3				
4				

Figure 12.2 An example continuing professional development recording proforma for learning starting at reflection.

Adapted from General Pharmaceutical Council. *Plan and Record: A Guide to the GPhC's Requirements for Undertaking and Recording Continuing Professional Development.* July 2011 (version ii). © GPhC 2011.

ACTION

When did you complete the activities outlined in your plan?

Record the date on which you completed the activities that you chose from your plan. The number in the option column should correspond to the options you selected in the question above.

Option	Description of what you did	Date completed

What have you learnt?

Describe what specific skill, knowledge, attitudes and/or behaviours you've gained as a result of your learning. This may be different to what you originally set out to learn.

EVALUATION

To what extent did you learn what you set out to learn at the start of this CPD cycle?

You may find it useful to revisit the 'Reflection' section and decide on what you originally wanted to learn before you decide to what extent you've achieved this learning.

Fully ❑   Partly ❑   Not at all ❑

If you ticked 'fully' or 'partly', give an example of how you've applied what you learnt to your practice

Putting learning into practice is a good way to prove that you've actually learnt what you set out to. It's not enough just to write about what you intend to do.

If you ticked 'fully' or 'partly', describe what have been, or what will be, the benefits to your practice.

If you ticked 'partly' or 'not at all', describe what it is you still have to learn.

You may find it useful to revisit the 'Reflection' section and check on what it is you originally wanted to learn before you describe what it is you still need to learn.

If you ticked 'partly' or 'not at all', explain why you think you didn't achieve your learning.

You may find it useful to revisit the 'Reflection' and 'Planning' sections to work out why you didn't achieve everything you set out to learn. It's all right for you not to have achieved all of your learning, but it is important that you explain why.

Figure 12.2 (continued)

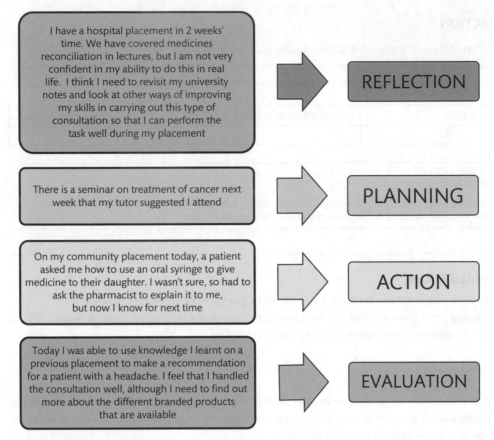

Figure 12.3 Examples of learning opportunities and where they fit in the continuing professional development cycle.

identified but because their tutor has suggested that they attend. However, this can still be valid CPD, as long as what they learn is relevant to their role.

The 'starting at action' example shows learning that has not been planned in advance; a situation has occurred, and, during the course of this, the student has learnt something new which will be beneficial in the future.

In the final example, 'starting at evaluation', the student has applied some prior learning and considered the benefits of this learning. They have also identified a further learning need, which they can take forward into a new learning cycle, starting at 'reflection'.

Hints and tips for writing continuing professional development entries

Reflection

- Choose your learning objective carefully. If your learning objective isn't right, then it is likely that the rest of your CPD entry won't quite work either.
- Be clear about what you want to learn—you should choose a specific skill, knowledge, or behaviour to develop.

- Take care not to choose a learning objective that is too broad, as this will be difficult to achieve.
- Ensure that the topic of what you want to learn is relevant to you and your practice (now or in the future)—is it something that will make you a better pharmacy student or pharmacist of the future?
- Think about what it was that prompted you to choose this subject as something to learn more about. Was it a particular event, or talking to a colleague, or something that you were personally interested in?

Planning

- Choose a realistic timescale for your learning. You will need to give yourself enough time to undertake the learning activities, while ensuring that you complete your learning in time to use it when you need it.
- Think about the importance of what you are planning to learn. Consider this from a range of viewpoints—for example, its importance to you, to patients, or your colleagues/ peers. As mentioned earlier, if it is of low importance, you may wish to revisit the topic you have chosen.
- Remember to consider a range of ways in which you might achieve the learning need that you have identified—you don't necessarily need to undertake all of these. For each, think about the advantages and disadvantages, as this will help you to decide which activities to choose to take forward.

Action

- Clearly describe the activities that you undertook.
- If you read a textbook or a journal article, include the reference for it, so that someone else reading your record could identify the source of information that you used. If you used a website, include the website address and the date that you accessed it.
- If you shadowed, or had a discussion with, a colleague, give some detail about who they were—this will help to show why they were an appropriate source of information. It may not be appropriate to give their name, for confidentiality reasons; in this case, you could perhaps give their job title/role instead.
- Give a clear description of what you learnt, whether that is new knowledge, a skill, or a change in behaviour.
- Don't panic if what you ended up learning was not what you intended to learn! Sometimes things change as we go through the learning process. You will have the opportunity to discuss this in your evaluation.

Evaluation

- Think about the extent to which you achieved what you set out to achieve—fully, partly, or not at all.
- Where possible, give an example of a situation in which you have used what you have learnt. Ideally, this will be a situation involving patient care, but other examples include

being able to pass on your learning to others (e.g. through teaching), or completing a piece of work or other task.

- Also consider what benefit this learning has had for you and others—compare this with what you anticipated the benefits to be during the planning stage.
- If you only partly achieved what you set out to, or feel that you didn't achieve anything at all, think about why this might have been, what you still need to learn, and what you might do next in order to do this.

Portfolio of evidence

Alongside your records of CPD, you may decide to keep a portfolio of evidence—a folder in which you keep documents relating to learning activities that you have undertaken. These documents might include certificates of attendance for workshops or seminars, handouts from lectures, the agenda from a meeting that you have attended, or an email from a colleague regarding an activity that you have undertaken. How you put your portfolio together is a matter of personal preference, but you should aim to do this in a way which makes it easy for you to locate individual documents in the future should you need to. If you are required to maintain a portfolio as one of the assessments for your course, ensure that you have followed the instructions given to you by your course tutor. For documents that relate to a specific CPD entry, you may wish to add some form of numbering or referencing system to make it easy to match them up. Keeping a portfolio may also be useful for job applications in the future.

 ### Real-practice examples

Boxes 12.1 and 12.2 give two examples of CPD entries; Box 12.1 is an entry that might be made by a pharmacy student; Box 12.2 is an example of a real CPD entry, written by a hospital pharmacist. Hopefully, these will give you an indication of how you might make a start on completing your own CPD records.

 Key points

- CPD is usually thought of as a cycle of learning, starting at reflection, then moving on to planning, taking action, then evaluating what has been learnt. As you complete one cycle of CPD, you may find that you are led on to another, as you identify a new learning need that you were not previously aware of.
- The detail of the regulator's requirement for pharmacists conducting CPD may change in future, perhaps with more of a focus on demonstrating a broader fitness to practice. However, the importance of CPD will remain in ensuring that pharmacists are able to maintain a high standard of patient care.
- Choosing an appropriate learning objective is key—it should be clear, specific, and relevant to your role.
- Learning can be achieved through many ways, so try to make use of all the learning opportunities that are available to you.

Box 12.1

Name of entry: Giving a presentation

REFLECTION

> This entry has a specific learning objective, with a clear reason for addressing it.

What do you want to learn?

I want to learn how to give a successful oral presentation of a patient case study.

How did you identify what you needed to learn?

As part of my Part 3 clinical module, I have to deliver a presentation about a patient with heart failure. I find that giving presentations makes me feel nervous and I feel unsure about how to structure the presentation so that my message gets across to the audience clearly, and I present well.

How is this learning relevant to the **safe** and effective practice of pharmacy and your own job role/future career as a pharmacist?

It is important for pharmacists to be able to communicate information in a clear and easy-to-understand manner. The skills that I learn now will therefore be helpful in the future.

PLANNING

> The timescale is appropriate and realistic in relation to when the learning needs to be completed by. A range of learning activities has been considered.

When will you need to have achieved this learning? In 1 month.

Why is this learning important to you and your practice?

This learning will help me to perform well in this assessment. As a pharmacist in the future, it is likely that I will have to give presentations on a range of topics, so learning how to present effectively now will help me in my future career.

What might you need to do in order to achieve this learning?

Option	Description of what you plan to do	Advantages	Disadvantages	Select (√ or ×)
1	Read the assessment handbook	Specifies the requirements for the assessment	Doesn't give information on how to manage the presentation, e.g. dealing with nerves, etc.	√
2	Read Chapter 6 of *Successful Learning in Pharmacy*	Gives advice and tips on how to structure and deliver presentations	Does not contain the marking criteria for this specific assessment	√
3	Watch a YouTube video on giving presentations	More interesting than reading	There are lots of different videos available and it is difficult to know which are reliable and of good quality	

ACTION

When did you complete the activities outlined in your plan?

Option	Description of what you did	Date completed
1	Read the assessment handbook for module PH3PM	Date
2	Read Chapter 6 of *Successful Learning in Pharmacy* (Donyai P, Grant D, Patel N. *Successful Learning in Pharmacy*. Oxford: Oxford University Press; 2017).	Date

What have you learnt?

I have learnt how to structure a case study presentation, using a mind map to help me ensure that I include all of the relevant information about the case. I have learnt that good preparation is important in reducing nerves when giving a presentation and I have learnt some tips to help ensure that my presentation goes well.

EVALUATION

To what extent did you learn what you set out to learn at the start of this CPD cycle?

Fully √   Partly ❑   Not at all ❑

If you ticked 'fully' or 'partly', give an example of how you've applied what you learnt to your practice.

I gave my presentation on a patient with heart failure. Although I was nervous, I felt this less than last time I gave a presentation and was glad that I had prepared well as it helped my confidence. The presentation seemed to flow well and I was able to answer questions that were posed at the end of the talk. I received a good mark and positive feedback from the tutor.

If you ticked 'fully' or 'partly', describe what have been, or what will be, the benefits to your practice.

I now feel more confident when giving presentations and think that this will develop further as I gain more experience. This will be useful in my final year project presentation and also in the future, when giving presentations in my career as a pharmacist.

Box 12.2

Name of entry: Treatment of Urinary Tract Infections (UTIs)

REFLECTION

What do you want to learn?

> I want to learn the antibiotic choices that can be used for treatment of UTIs within the guidelines used at my hospital, particularly for patients in special groups (e.g. renal impairment).

How did you identify what you needed to learn?

> A patient on the ward I was covering was prescribed nitrofurantoin for a UTI. This was according to protocol, but the patient had renal impairment, making the nitrofurantoin inappropriate. Although I knew what drugs could be used to treat UTIs, I was not familiar with the hospital's specific guidance.

How is this learning relevant to the safe and effective practice of pharmacy and your own job role/future career as a pharmacist?

> This learning will help me to screen prescriptions for patients with UTIs more effectively and give advice to medical staff when asked.

PLANNING

When will you need to have achieved this learning? In 1 week.

Why is this learning important to you and your practice?

> I will be able to make more complete interventions in situations where the first-line treatment for UTI is not appropriate and ensure that patients receive treatment as recommended by the microbiology team. I will be able to give better advice to medical staff.

What might you need to do in order to achieve this learning?

Option	Description of what you plan to do	Advantages	Disadvantages	Select (√ or ×)
1	Read the hospital guidelines	Give a quick overview of the recommended treatments and are quite clear	Only give first- and second-line treatments and do not take account of special groups of patients	√
2	Speak to the specialist pharmacist	The specialist pharmacist was involved with producing the guideline and will be able to give more in-depth information and rationale for choices	They are busy and not always available	√

ACTION

When did you complete the activities outlined in your plan?

Option	Description of what you did	Date completed
1	Read the hospital's 'Guideline for the Management of Urinary Tract Infections'	Date
2	Spoke to the antimicrobial specialist pharmacist	Date

What have you learnt?

> I have learnt that co-amoxiclav is first-line treatment for UTIs, with nitrofurantoin second line in patients allergic to penicillin. Where patients are renally impaired, cefalexin 500 mg TDS may be used (depending on severity of penicillin allergy) or, if not appropriate, then ciprofloxacin is the last choice (owing to risk of *Clostridium difficile*-associated diarrhoea).

EVALUATION

To what extent did you learn what you set out to learn at the start of this CPD cycle?

Fully √   Partly ❑   Not at all ❑

If you ticked 'fully' or 'partly', give an example of how you've applied what you learnt to your practice.

> After I had completed my learning, another patient was admitted to the ward with a UTI. The patient was elderly and had renal impairment. I was asked by one of the junior doctors on the ward to recommend a suitable antibiotic and I was able to provide appropriate information in accordance with the hospital's guidance. The doctor thanked me for my help and the patient was successfully treated.

If you ticked 'fully' or 'partly', describe what have been, or what will be, the benefits to your practice.

> I am now better able to make interventions regarding appropriate treatment of UTIs, in accordance with the Trust's guidelines.

 Further reading and references

The General Pharmaceutical Council has prepared a document describing their requirements for pharmacists completing CPD. It also provides some pointers for successful CPD records. Plan and Record: A Guide to the GPhC's Requirements for Undertaking and Recording Continuing Professional Development [downloadable PDF document]. Available from: http://www.pharmacyregulation.org/sites/default/files/gphc_plan_and_record_dec_2015_0.pdf [Accessed 6 December 2016].

The Royal Pharmaceutical Society (RPS) also provides guidance regarding CPD. See: http://www. rpharms.com/development/continuing-professional-development.asp [Accessed 30 August 2015]. Note that some parts of this website are only available to members of the RPS.

Department of Health. Allied Health Professions Project: Demonstrating Competence Through Continuing Professional Development Final Report. London: Department of Health; 2003.

Royal Pharmaceutical Society. *RPS Foundation Pharmacy Framework* [downloadable PDF document]. Available from: https://www.rpharms.com/development-files/foundation-pharmacy-framework---final.pdf [Accessed 30 May 2016].

Index